DOCUMENTATION & THE NURSING PROCESS

DOCUMENTATION & THE NURSING PROCESS

Lois White, RN, PhD

Former Chairperson and Professor
Department of Vocational Nurse Education
Del Mar College
Corpus Christi, Texas

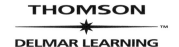

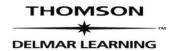

THOMSON

TM

DELMAR LEARNING

Documentation & the Nursing Process

Healthcare Publishing Director: William Brottmiller	**Acquisitions Editor:** Matthew Filimonov	**Channel Manager:** Jennifer McAvey
Executive Editor: Cathy L. Esperti	**Editorial Assistant:** Patricia Osborn	**Production Editor:** James Zayicek
	Executive Marketing Manager: Dawn F. Gerrain	

COPYRIGHT © 2003 by Delmar, a division of Thomson Learning, Inc. Thomson Learning™ is a trademark used herein under license.

Printed in Canada

1 2 3 4 5 XXX 07 06 05 04 03 02

For more information, contact Delmar Learning
5 Maxwell Drive
Clifton Park, NY 12065

Or find us on the World Wide Web at http://www.delmar.com

Library of Congress Cataloging-in-Publication Data
White, Lois.
    Documentation & the nursing process / Lois White.
        p. cm.
    Includes index.
    ISBN 0-7668-5009-9
    1. Nursing records--Handbooks, manuals, etc. I. Title.
RT50 . W457 2002
651.5'04261--dc21   2002067673

Notice to the Reader

Contents

Preface

Documentation & the Nursing Process was developed following requests from the faculty of several nursing programs for a small book on documentation that students could carry with them in the clinical area for quick reference. Documentation has always been an important aspect of nursing; however, with the increases in the number of lawsuits filed against health care personnel and agencies, documentation has become a critical aspect of nursing. In this book, the mechanics and legal aspects of documentation are explained, as well as, the different types of documentation. Examples are provided.

Organization

Documentation & the Nursing Process is divided into two units with six chapters in each.

Unit 1 is a review of the nursing process.

Chapter 1, Nursing Process, provides an overview of the nursing process and how it relates to critical thinking, problem solving, decision making, and holistic care.

Chapter 2, Assessment, describes the purpose of assessment and how to collect and validate data, and how to organize, interpret and document the collected data.

Chapter 3, Diagnosis, discusses how nursing diagnosis and medical diagnosis are different, the components of a nursing diagnosis, how to write a nursing diagnosis statement, the various types of nursing diagnoses, and collaborative problems. Many examples are provided.

Chapter 4, Planning and Outcome Identification, explains how nursing diagnoses are prioritized, and outcomes identified, the difference between goals and outcomes, the categories of nursing interventions, and the recording of the nursing care plan.

Chapter 5, Implementation, discusses the requirements for effective implementation, the various types of nursing interventions, and the documenting as well as reporting of interventions.

Chapter 6, Evaluation, demonstrates how evaluation is fundamental to each aspect of the nursing process and in determining whether or not goals were met. A brief description of nursing audit is also included.

Unit 2, Documentation, discusses the reasons for documenting, the principles and methods, various forms used, trends, and reporting.

Chapter 7, Documentation as Communication, identifies the purposes of documentation including communication, education, research, and reimbursement. Legal and practice standards are also discussed.

Chapter 8, Principles of Effective Documentation, emphasizes the importance of following the nursing process. The elements of effective documentation are explained and examples provided.

Chapter 9, Methods of Documentation, shares a description and examples of various methods of documentation including narrative, source-oriented, problem-oriented, PIE, and focus charting, charting by exception, computerized charting, point-of-care charting, and critical pathway.

Chapter 10, Forms for Recording Data, provides an explanation of the use of Kardex, flow sheets, nurses' progress notes, and discharge summary. Many examples are included.

Chapter 11, Trends in Documentation, introduces the student to a data set, nursing interventions classification, and nursing outcomes classification, and how nursing diagnoses are evolving.

Chapter 12, Reporting, develops the idea that information important enough to report should also be documented. Various types of reporting are discussed including summary reports, walking rounds, telephone reports and orders, and incident reports.

Features

Each chapter opens with *Learning Objectives* to guide the reader's learning. *Key Terms* are listed to identify important terms in the chapter. *Professional Tip* and *Community/Home Health Care* boxes highlight important information. A *Summary,* multiple choice *Review Questions,* and *Critical Thinking Questions* at the end of each chapter help the student remember and use the material presented. *Web Flash!* boxes guide the student to the Internet for current information related to chapter content. A *Case Study* at the end of Chapter 6 helps the student see how the individual aspects of the nursing process fit together. The *References/Suggested Readings* and *Resources* provide access to the source of material in the chapters and places to obtain additional material. The Appendices provide (A) a listing of NANDA Nursing Diagnoses; (B) Abbreviations, Acronyms, and Symbols, and (C) Answers to Review Questions. A Glossary and Index are also included.

Acknowledgments

My sincere thanks to Matt Filimonov, acquisitions editor, Patricia Osborn, editorial assistant, and to the entire team at Delmar Learning who have worked to make this text a reality. To the reviewers, thank you for the time spent critically reading the manuscript and for the pertinent remarks and helpful suggestions. Thank you to all who worked on this text.

About the Author

Lois Elain Wacker White earned a diploma in nursing from Memorial Hospital School of Nursing, Springfield, Illinois; an Associate degree in Science from Del Mar College, Corpus Christi, Texas; a Bachelor of Science in Nursing from Texas A & I University-Corpus Christi, Corpus Christi, Texas; a Master of Science in Education from Corpus Christi State University, Corpus Christi, Texas; and a Doctor of Philosophy degree in educational administration–community college from the University of Texas, Austin, Texas.

She has taught at Del Mar College, Corpus Christi, Texas in both the Associate Degree Nursing program and the Vocational Nursing program. For 14 years she was also chairperson of the Department of Vocational Nurse Education. Dr. White has taught fundamentals of nursing, nutrition, mental health/mental illness, medical-surgical nursing, and maternal/newborn nursing. Her professional career has also included 15 years of clinical practice.

Dr. White has served on the Nursing Education Advisory Committee of the Texas Board of Nurse Examiners and the Texas Board of Vocational Nurse Examiners, which developed competencies expected of graduates from each level of nursing. She maintains membership in the Texas Association of Vocational Nurse Educators, Sigma Theta Tau International, American Nurses Association, and the National League for Nursing.

Dr. White has been listed in *Who's Who in American Nursing*. She currently serves on the Vocational Nursing Financial Aid Advisory Committee for the Texas Higher Education Coordinating Board.

REVIEWERS

Anita G. Kinser, MSN, RNC
Assistant Professor of Nursing
Riverside Community College
Riverside, California

Mary S. Lewin, RN, BSN, MSEd
Licensed Practical Nursing Instructor
Orleans Career and Technical Center
Medina, New York

Karen S. March
Assistant Professor of Nursing
University of Pittsburgh at Bradford
Bradford, Pennsylvania

Ester Gonzales, RN, MSN, MSEd
Del Mar College
Corpus Christi, Texas

UNIT
1

Nursing Process

CHAPTER

1

NURSING
PROCESS

INTRODUCTION

The nursing process is a systematic method of planning and providing care to clients. It is the basis for accurate, complete documentation required to meet legal standards as well as the standards of care identified in the state nursing practice acts and by the Joint Commission on Accreditation of Healthcare Organizations (JCAHO). Therefore, it is fitting to begin a text on documentation with a review of the nursing process. Use of the nursing process allows nurses to communicate their roles in planning and executing client-centered activities to clients, their families, and other health care professionals. It is a process that encourages orderly thought, analysis, and planning when working with clients to decide those things that need to be done. The nursing process consists of five steps: assessment, diagnosis, planning and outcome identification, implementation, and evaluation.

This chapter presents information about the historical development of the nursing process. A discussion on the way the nurse uses critical thinking in each step of the nursing process is included. The relationship of the nursing process to problem solving, decision making, and collaboration is also discussed.

HISTORICAL PERSPECTIVE

Lydia Hall first referred to nursing as a "process" in a 1955 journal article, yet the term *nursing process* was not widely used until the late 1960s (Edelman & Mandle, 2001). Referring to the nursing process as a series of steps, Johnson (1959), Orlando (1961), and Wiedenbach (1963) further developed this description of nursing. At that time, the nursing process involved only three steps: assessment, planning, and evaluation. In their 1967 book *The Nursing Process*, Yura and Walsh identified four steps in the nursing process:

- Assessing
- Planning
- Implementing
- Evaluating

Fry (1953) first used the term *nursing diagnosis*, but it was not until 1974, after the first meeting of the group now called the North American Nursing Diagnosis Association (NANDA), that nursing diagnosis was added as a separate and distinct step in the nursing process. Prior to this, nursing diagnosis had been included as a natural conclusion to the first step, assessment. Currently, the steps in the nursing process are:

- Assessment
- Diagnosis
- Planning and outcome identification
- Implementation
- Evaluation

OVERVIEW OF THE NURSING PROCESS

A **process** is a series of steps or acts that lead to accomplishment of some goal or purpose. According to Bevis, "processes have three characteristics: (1) inherent purpose, (2) internal organization, and (3) infinite creativity" (1989). These characteristics can be applied to the nursing process. The **nursing process** is a systematic method of planning and providing care to clients. The purpose is to provide client care that is individualized, holistic, effective, and efficient. Although the steps of the nursing process build on each other, they are not linear. Each step overlaps with the previous and subsequent steps (Figure 1-1).

The nursing process is dynamic and requires creativity in its application. Although the steps remain the same in each client situation, the application and results will differ. The nursing process is designed to be used with clients throughout the life span and in any care setting. It is also a basic organizing system for the National Council Licensure Examination for both

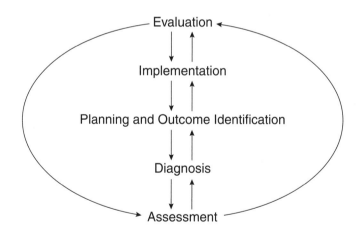

NURSING PROCESS

Figure 1-1 Five Components of the Nursing Process: Assessment, Diagnosis, Planning and Outcome Identification, Implementation, and Evaluation. The arrows going down represent revisions.

practical/vocational nurses (NCLEX-PN)® and registered nurses (NCLEX-RN)®. The steps of the nursing process are specifically mentioned in *Nursing Practice Standards for the Licensed Practical/Vocational Nurse*, National Federation of Licensed Practical Nurses (NFLPN) (1996) and in *Standards of Clinical Nursing Practice*, American Nurses Association (ANA) (1991).

 PROFESSIONAL TIP

The Nursing Process
- Rather than being linear, the nursing process involves overlapping steps.
- The steps are explained one after the other for ease of understanding, but in actual practice, there may not be a definite beginning or ending to each step.
- Work in one step may begin before work in the preceding step is completed.

THE NURSING PROCESS AND CRITICAL THINKING

A number of skills are required of nurses in their use of the nursing process as a framework for providing client care. One important skill is critical thinking. Critical thinkers ask questions, evaluate evidence, identify assumptions, examine alternatives, and seek to understand various points of view.

Critical thinking is a skill that can be learned, just as other skills are learned. The skill of critical thinking is important and useful in all aspects of a person's life and is an especially vital tool for the nurse with regard to the nursing process. Critical thinkers develop a questioning attitude and delve into situations in order to seek possible explanations for what is happening. Examples of questions that the nurse as critical thinker might ask at each step in the nursing process are listed in Table 1-1.

Assumptions are those beliefs or attitudes that one takes for granted in a situation that requires action or resolution; they are the things that one accepts as "given." Assumptions are the implicit views one uses to filter and make sense of everyday

Table 1-1   USE OF CRITICAL THINKING WITH THE NURSING PROCESS

STEP OF NURSING PROCESS	SAMPLE CRITICAL THINKING QUESTIONS
Assessment	What data are necessary to prevent, anticipate, or detect health problems? What data are necessary to manage or eliminate a client's health problems? From what other sources can data be obtained? How does the client view his health situation? How efficient is care delivery? What assumptions or biases does the nurse have?
Diagnosis	How can the data be put together and analyzed? Are there any gaps in the data? What health problems can be identified? What are the underlying causes of or risk factors for the health problems? What are the client's strengths and resources? Which satisfactory aspects of the client's health could be improved?
Planning and Outcome Identification	What are the specific desired outcomes for this client? What interventions will detect or prevent health problems? Which interventions will manage the client's health problems? What interventions will promote optimum wellness and independence for the client? How can the desired outcomes be achieved in a cost-effective, timely manner? Who is best qualified to carry out the interventions? How much does the client wish to be involved?

(continues)

Table 1-1 USE OF CRITICAL THINKING WITH THE NURSING PROCESS *continued*	
STEP OF NURSING PROCESS	**SAMPLE CRITICAL THINKING QUESTIONS**
Implementation	How ready is the health care giver to perform the interventions? What are the critical steps of this intervention? How can the intervention be altered to meet this client's needs yet maintain principles of safety? How does the client respond during and after the intervention? What is to be documented to monitor the client's progress toward the goals and outcomes?
Evaluation	Were the specific desired goals and outcomes met? If all were met, can these goals and outcomes be eliminated? If not met, how should the plan be modified (revised)? If revision of the plan, goals, or outcomes is necessary, what ongoing, continuous assessments (data) are identified? Were assumptions or biases missed that affected the interventions? What other nursing diagnosis(es) may be appropriate? What additional outcomes and interventions should be considered?

experiences. Cause-and-effect relationships are understood within the context of these assumptions. Assumptions both are related to one's point of view and influence the way one looks at things.

Bias is a personal judgment or inclination. It can be manifested in either of two ways. According to one interpretation of bias, a person's point of view causes that person to be more observant about certain things. Another interpretation of bias holds that a person is blind to or unwilling to consider weaknesses in his own point of view. Critical thinkers attempt to be aware of both interpretations of bias and to avoid the latter.

Alfaro-LeFevre (1999) suggests three questions to ask when making decisions about managing client's health problems:

1. Does the facility have specific guidelines or policies for the care of this specific situation?
2. Are there national practice guidelines relating to this particular problem?
3. To what degree do these standards apply to the specific client's situation?

THE NURSING PROCESS AND PROBLEM SOLVING

The steps in the nursing process and in problem solving are similar. People use problem solving in their daily lives. With the problem-solving method, a problem is acknowledged, information is gathered, a specific problem is identified, a plan for solving the problem is developed, the plan is carried out, and results of the plan are evaluated. Problem solving, however, is frequently based on incomplete data, and plans are sometimes based on guesses. Conversely, the nursing process, which is used by nurses to identify and make decisions about client needs, is a systematic and scientifically based process that requires the use of many cognitive and psychomotor skills. Table 1-2 compares the nursing process and the problem-solving method.

THE NURSING PROCESS AND DECISION MAKING

Nurses make decisions every day. It is important that those decisions be the best decisions possible, that they be based on reliable information, and that they be made with as much critical thought as possible. Nurses make decisions at each step of the nursing process. Through a process of problem solving, one arrives at the point at which decisions can be made. The nursing process is the specific problem-solving method used by

Table 1-2	COMPARISON OF THE PROBLEM-SOLVING METHOD AND THE NURSING PROCESS

PROBLEM-SOLVING METHOD	NURSING PROCESS
Acknowledge a problem	Assessment
Gather information	Assessment
Identify the problem	Diagnosis
Develop a plan	Planning and outcome identification
Carry out plan	Implementation
Evaluate results	Evaluation

nurses to arrive at the point at which decisions about client care can be made.

Because the nursing process is a dynamic, circular, and fluid process, decisions must be made at many points as the nurse implements the various steps. Each of these decisions, resulting from critical thought and problem-solving strategies, leads to the determination of appropriate nursing interventions for the client.

THE NURSING PROCESS AND HOLISTIC CARE

Nurses bring to each client situation a broad knowledge base. The theoretical base of nursing knowledge comes from many different fields, including the natural sciences, behavioral sciences, social sciences, arts and humanities, and nursing science. This broad knowledge base allows the nurse to interact with the client from a holistic viewpoint. Each nurse–client interaction adds to the client database and allows for individualized planning and care. The nursing process assists the nurse in determining client responses to situations, and critical-thinking and decision-making skills allow the nurse to prioritize client needs and decide which person can best meet certain client needs.

Referral and collaboration among nurses and other health care professionals contribute to optimal achievement of client goals.

In some settings, the traditional nursing care plan formulated solely by nurses has been replaced by plans that are developed by a multidisciplinary team and referred to as critical pathways. **Critical pathways** are comprehensive, standard plans of care for specific case situations. Included in these plans are nursing interventions, medical interventions, interventions from other team members, specific client outcomes, and time lines for those outcomes. Because the nurse has a broad base of knowledge, the nurse is often the person who manages the care of the client through these critical pathways.

SUMMARY

- The nursing process is an organized method of planning and delivering nursing care. It is composed of five steps: assessment, diagnosis, planning and outcome identification, implementation, and evaluation.
- Critical thinking is an integral part of each step of the nursing process.
- Problem-solving, and decision-making skills are important in the use of the nursing process.

Review Questions

1. Which of the following statements would describe the nursing process?
   a. It is a linear, static procedure.
   b. It is a circular, dynamic process.
   c. It is a hierarchy of steps to plan client care.
   d. It is a long, detailed form to be filled out for each client.

2. Currently, the steps in the nursing process include diagnosis, assessment, evaluation, planning and outcome identification and:
   a. intervention.
   b. implementation.
   c. critical thinking.
   d. internal organization.

3. The steps of the nursing process are specifically mentioned in the American Nurses Association's *Standards of Care* and in the:
  a. National League for Nursing's *Standards of Care*.
  b. American Federation of RNs and LP/VNs *Standards of Care*.
  c. National Federation of Licensed Practical Nurses *Standards of Care*.
  d. National Association of Practical Nurses Education and Service's *Standards of Care*.

4. The nurse knows that a collaborative nursing diagnosis is appropriate when:
  a. the family wishes to care for the client.
  b. the client assists the nurse in caring for himself.
  c. two or more nurses must work together to care for the client.
  d. the client's health situation has commonly occurring complications for which the nurses monitor.

Critical Thinking Questions

1. How is critical thinking related to the nursing process?

2. How are the nursing process and problem-solving the same? How are they different?

 WEB FLASH!

- Can you find specific sites or resources dealing with the nursing process?
- Do the resources listed for this chapter also have web sites? What types of information do they provide?
- What resources on the Internet are available for nurses needing assistance with the nursing process or nursing diagnosis?

References/Suggested Readings

Alfaro-LeFevre, R. (1998). *Applying nursing process* (4th ed.). Philadelphia: Lippincott Williams & Wilkins.

Alfaro-LeFevre, R. (1999). *Critical thinking in nursing: A practical approach* (2nd ed.). Philadelphia: W. B. Saunders Company.

American Nurses Association. (1991). *Standards of nursing practice.* Kansas City, MO: Author.

Bevis, E. O. (1989). *Curriculum building in nursing: A process* (3rd ed., Publication No. 15-2277). New York: National League for Nursing.

Carpenito, L. J. (2000). *Nursing diagnosis: Application to clinical practice* (8th ed.). Philadelphia: Lippincott Williams & Wilkins.

DeLaune, S., & Ladner, P. (2002). *Fundamentals of nursing: Standards & practice* (2nd ed.). Albany, NY: Delmar.

Edelman, C. L., & Mandle, C. L. (2001). *Health promotion throughout the lifespan* (6th ed.). St. Louis, MO: Mosby.

Fry, V. S. (1953). The creative approach to nursing. *AJN, 53*(3), 301–302.

Gardner, P. (2002). *Nursing process.* Albany, NY: Delmar.

Gordon, M. (2000). *Manual of nursing diagnoses* (9th ed.). St. Louis, MO: Mosby.

Johnson, D. (1959). A philosophy for nursing diagnosis. *Nursing Outlook, 7,* 198–200.

National Federation of Licensed Practical Nurses (NFLPN). (1996). *Nursing practice standards for the licensed practical/vocational nurse.* Garner, NC: Author.

North American Nursing Diagnosis Association (NANDA). (2001). *Nursing diagnoses: Definitions & classifications 2001–2002.* Philadelphia: Author.

Orem, D. E., Taylor, S. G., & Renpenning, K. (2001). *Nursing: Concepts of practice* (6th ed.). St. Louis, MO: Mosby.

Orlando, I. (1961). *The dynamic nurse–patient relationship.* New York: Putnam.

Paul, R. W. (1995). *Critical thinking: How to prepare students for a rapidly changing world.* Santa Rosa, CA: Foundation for Critical Thinking.

Seaback, W. (2001). *Nursing process: Concepts & application.* Albany, NY: Delmar.

White, L. (2001). *Foundations of nursing: Caring for the whole person.* Albany, NY: Delmar.

White, L. (2002). *Basic nursing: Foundations of skills & concepts.* Albany, NY: Delmar.

Wiedenbach, E. (1963). The helping art of nursing. *AJN, 63*(11), 54–57.

Wilkinson, J. M. (2001). *Nursing process and critical thinking* (3rd ed.). Englewood Cliffs, NJ: Prentice Hall.

Yoder Wise, P. S. (1998). *Leading and managing in nursing* (2nd ed.). St. Louis, MO: Mosby.

Yura, H., & Walsh, M. B. (1967). *The nursing process.* Washington, DC: Catholic University of America Press.

CHAPTER 2

ASSESSMENT

INTRODUCTION

Assessment is the first step in the nursing process and includes the systematic collection, verification, organization, interpretation, and documentation of client data. It is a very important step because the completeness and correctness of the information obtained in this step are directly related to the accuracy of the steps that follow. Assessment involves several steps:

- Collecting data from a variety of sources
- Validating the data

- Organizing the data
- Interpreting the data
- Documenting the data

PURPOSE OF ASSESSMENT

The purpose of assessment is to establish a **database**, a foundation of information, concerning a client's physical, psychosocial, and emotional health in order to identify health-promoting behaviors as well as actual and/or potential health problems. Through assessment, the nurse ascertains the client's functional abilities and the absence or presence of dysfunction. The client's normal activities of daily living and lifestyle patterns are also assessed. Identification of the client's strengths provides the nurse and other members of the treatment team information about the skills, abilities, and behaviors the client has available to promote the treatment and recovery process. The assessment phase also offers an opportunity for the nurse to form a therapeutic interpersonal relationship with the client. During assessment, the client is provided an opportunity to discuss health care concerns and goals with the nurse.

Database

The **database** is information about the client prior to entering the health care system. It is the information foundation (database) against which changes in the client's health status are measured. That is, is there improvement, deterioration, or no change? The database is generally collected upon admission through a physical examination and a complete health history including a review of physical and psychosocial aspects of the client's health, the client's perception of health, the presence of health risk factors, and the client's coping patterns.

COLLECTING DATA

Data are collected by using various types of assessments and from a variety of sources. The collected data are either subjective or objective.

Types of Assessment

The type and scope of information needed for assessment are usually determined by the health care setting and needs of the client. Three types of assessment are comprehensive, focused, and ongoing. Although a comprehensive assessment is most desirable in initially determining a client's need for nursing care, time limitations or special circumstances may dictate the need for abbreviated data collection, such as the focused assessment. The assessment database can then be expanded after the initial focused assessment, and data should be updated through ongoing assessment.

Comprehensive Assessment A **comprehensive assessment** gathers client information through a complete health history, physical examination, a review of psychosocial aspects of the client's health, the client's perception of health, the presence of health risk factors, and the client's coping patterns. It is usually completed upon admission to a health care agency (Figure 2-1).

Focused Assessment A **focused assessment** is an assessment that is limited in scope in order to concentrate on a particular need or health care concern or on potential health care risks. Focused assessments are not as detailed as comprehensive assessments and are often used in health care agencies where short stays are anticipated (e.g., outpatient surgery centers and emergency departments), in specialty areas such as labor and delivery, in mental health settings, or for the purpose of screening for specific problems or risk factors (e.g., well-child clinics).

Ongoing Assessment Systematic follow-up is required when problems are identified during a comprehensive or focused assessment. An **ongoing assessment** is an assessment that includes systematic monitoring and observation related to

 COMMUNITY/HOME HEALTH CARE

Ongoing Assessment
- In the home, ongoing assessment may involve specific questions to elicit specific information.
- Clients are more comfortable and feel in charge in their own homes as opposed to a health care facility.
- The client may have a tendency to spend a lot of time telling stories about past medical problems and treatment, as opposed to providing information relevant to the situation at hand (Humphrey, 1998).

DATE:	REASON FOR HOSPITALIZATION (E.R. TRIAGE/DIAGNOSIS)	
TIME:		

MODE OF ARRIVAL	ONSET OF SYMPTOMS (E.R. TRIAGE)	
Ambulance ☐		
Wheelchair ☐	PAST HISTORY: (Past Surgeries / Hospitalization) (E.R. TRIAGE)	
Stretcher ☐		
Ambulatory ☐		
	COMMENTS:	

VITAL SIGNS		HEALTH HISTORY		PERSON TO NOTIFY IN CASE OF EMERGENCY	
TEMP		✓ Only those conditions that patient has history or current condition			
PULSE		GLAUCOMA ☐	GASTRIC ULCERS ☐	NAME	
RESP		CANCER ☐	HEPATITIS ☐		
BP		LUNG DISEASE ☐	HIV DISEASE ☐		
	STATED	ASTHMA ☐	DIABETIC # OF YRS___	RELATIONSHIP	
HEIGHT	ACTUAL	KIDNEY DISEASE ☐	ANESTHESIA REACTION ☐		
	STATED	HEART DISEASE ☐	STROKE ☐		
WEIGHT	ACTUAL	PACEMAKER ☐	SEIZURE ☐	HAS POWER OF ATTORNEY FOR HEALTH CARE?	
ALLERGIES		HYPERTENSION ☐	TUBERCULOSIS ☐		
FOOD		ALCOHOL ☐	PSYCHIATRIC DX ☐	☐ YES ☐ NO	
LATEX ☐		SMOKING ☐	BLOOD TRANSFUSION ☐	TELEPHONE #	
OTHER		DRUGS ☐	IN PAST 10 YEARS		

DRUG ALLERGIES	REACTION	DATE
1.		
2.		
3.		
4.		
5.		

MEDICATIONS (E.R. MEDS)					ORGAN DONATION
Name	Dose	Freq	Reason	Last Dose	Do you want information on organ donation?
					YES ☐ NO ☐
					Referred to: ☐ Organ Transplant Alliance 887-6189
					PATIENT RIGHTS
					☐ Received copy of Patient Rights
					☐ Verbalizes understanding and ability to implement
					SIGNATURES:
					Completed by:_____
Meds Sent Home: YES ☐	NO ☐		N/A ☐		Entered by:_____

CHRISTUS SPOHN HEALTH SYSTEM

PATIENT ADMISSION
DATA BASE

2705318   NEW: 06/95
                           REVISED: 02/99.F10

(continues)

Figure 2-1 Patient Admission Data Base (Courtesy of CHRISTUS Spohn Health System, Corpus Christi, TX)

specific problems. This type of assessment allows the nurse to broaden the database or to confirm the validity of the data obtained during the initial assessment. Ongoing assessment is particularly important when problems have been identified and a plan of care has been implemented to address these problems. Systematic monitoring and observation allow the nurse to determine the response to nursing interventions and to identify any emerging problems.

FUNCTIONAL SCREENING (ADULT)

*Physical Therapy:	*Occupational Therapy	*Speech Therapy
0 pts = complete independence	0 pts = complete independence	0 pts = no identified problems
1 pt = recent onset of neurological problem	1 pt = acute decline in upper extremity function	2 pt = recent onset of swallowing problems
1 pt = recent onset of orthopedic problem		2 pt = recent onset of speech difficulty
1 pt = recent onset of problem with impaired mobility (ambulation, stair climbing, bed mobility, transferring)	1 pt = recent onset of a neurological or orthopedic problem	1 pt = recent neurological problem affecting ability to follow commands
2 pts = open wound or an acute burn	1 pt = recent onset of a problem causing a decrease in ADL function (Bathing, Dressing, Feeding Toileting)	2 pt = radical ENT surgery
____ TOTAL POINTS	____ TOTAL POINTS	____ TOTAL POINTS
* A Score of 2 or More Points Requires a Physical Therapy Screening.		
Physical Therapy Screening Requested	* A Score of 2 or More Points Requires an Occupational Therapy Screen.	* A Score of 2 or More Points Requires a Speech Therapy Screen.
☐ Yes ☐ No	Occupational Therapy Screening Requested	Speech Therapy Screening Requested
	☐ Yes ☐ No	☐ Yes ☐ No

PASTORAL CARE SCREEN	PATIENT INSTRUCTION CHECKLIST			
[ ] Would you like a special request sent for a visit from our chaplain?	☐ Signal Light	☐ Telephone	☐ Shower	☐ Dentures/Hearing Aid
[ ] Yes [ ] No	☐ Bed Controls	☐ Brochure	☐ T.V.	
[ ] If Yes, Send Request to Pastoral Care	☐ Light Controls	☐ Visiting Privileges	☐ I.D./Allergy Band On	
	☐ Bathroom	☐ Safety Precautions	☐ Pillow Speaker Placement	

PSYCHOSOCIAL/DISCHARGE PLANNING SCREEN

PSYCHOSOCIAL STATUS (circle all that apply)		LIVING ARRANGEMENT:		Current Resource Being		
				Utilized:	Yes	No
History of non-compliance impacting medical treatment	1	Family Unable to help/no known friends	2	Home Health	☐	☐
History alcohol/chemical abuse needing treatment	1	Age > 70 years lives alone	1	Provider	☐	☐
Suspected neglect/abuse	4	Patient admitted from other institution:	1	Private Sitter	☐	☐
Unsafe home environment (domestic violence/self-neglect)	4	___ SNF ___ NH		Meals on wheels	☐	☐
Prolonged confusion/disorientation	1	___ Rehab ___ Other Hospital		Hospice	☐	☐
Illness related anxiety impacting care	1	Patient is disabled	1	MHMR	☐	☐
Ineffective family coping patterns	1	Homeless or no address available	3	Adult Day Program	☐	☐
Recent loss of body limb	1			WIC Program	☐	☐
Terminal illness	4	ADMISSION STATUS:				
Suicide attempt/Ideation	4	Readmitted within 1 -30 days	1	DME AT HOME		
Significant Grief impacting care/treatment	1	Admitted through ER	1	☐ Oxygen ☐ Walker		
Teen Pregnancy (with high risk social factors)	2			☐ Wheelchair ☐ Trapeze		
Birth Anomalies or retardation	4	TOTAL OF ALL ____		☐ Hospital Bed		
Loss of Infant (fetal demise)	4	Low Risk = 0-2		☐ Bedside commode		
Adoption	4	Moderate Risk = 3 pts		Living with____		
Other: ____		High Risk = 4 or > pts				
		*HIGH RISK requires Social Services consult. Social Services notified ☐ Yes ☐ No				

VALUABLES BROUGHT WITH PATIENT TO HOSPITAL (SECURITY TAG)

Date:____

☐ Cane/Walker	☐ Bridgework no. of pieces ____	☐ Prothesis type ____	☐ Money (purse)	☐ Electric Razor
☐ Clocks	☐ Eyeglasses	☐ Hearing Aids L/R	☐ Wheelchair	☐ Clothing ____
☐ Dentures U/L	☐ Contact Lens	☐ Jewelry	☐ Radio	☐ Other ____
☐ Partial U/L	☐ Watches	☐ Money (billfold)	☐ T.V.	

I take entire responsibility for keeping in my possession the articles listed above. I am holding nothing in my possession which I have not declared here. I understand and agree that Christus Spohn Health System shall not be liable for the loss or damage to any money, jewelry, eyeglasses, dentures, hearing aids or other articles of value left in the care, custody and control of the patient or family/significant other.
It is understood and agreed that Christus Spohn Health System maintains a locked safe for money and valuables. The hospital shall not be liable for any of the patient's personal property that is not secured in the valuables storage envelope or in the hospital locked safe.

SIGNATURE OF PATIENT____
I have fully explained to this patient that Christus Spohn Health System takes no responsibility for articles retained by the patient.
SIGNATURE OF EMPLOYEE RECORDING ARTICLES____

Valuables given to: ____
VALUABLES STORAGE ENVELOPE: When valuables storage envelope is used, record the following information:
Valuables Storage Envelope Number ____ Date property received ____
Employee taking envelope to cashier ____ 2705318-2.F10 02/25/99

(continues)

Figure 2-1 *(continued)*

Sources of Data

Although data are collected from a variety of sources, the client should be considered the **primary source** of data (the major provider of information about a client). As much information as possible should be gathered from the client, using both interview techniques and physical examination skills. Data other than given by the client are considered **secondary**

RN ASSESSMENT: DATE:		TIME:		SIGNATURE:_____, RN

INSTRUCTION: 1. Complete physical assessment   3. Prioritize Problems
            2. Identify problems/nursing diagnosis for each system as appropriate   4. Enter problems for problem list in computer

SYSTEMS	YES	NO	COMMENTS	PROBLEM	SYSTEMS	PROBLEM
NEUROLOGICAL					CARDIOVASCULAR	
L.O.C.				☐ Thought processes,	Apical Rate [＿＿＿＿]	
• Alert				alteration in	Rhythm (circle one)	
• Drowsy				☐ Coping, ineffective	Regular	
• Comatose					Irregular	☐ Tissue
• Disoriented				☐ Communication,		perfusion
• Cooperative				impaired	On Cardiac Monitor: Yes No	alterations in
• Agitated					☐ ☐	
EYES				☐ Injury potential	If Yes: Rhythm _____	
• Pearl						☐ Comfort,
• Vision Normal				☐ Vision, impaired	Peripheral Pulses:	alterations in
• Prosthesis					Right Left	pain:
MOUTH				☐ Sensory, perception	Carotid ☐ ☐	
• Moist					Radial ☐ ☐	
• Lesions				☐ Other	Popliteal ☐ ☐	
• Teeth					Femoral ☐ ☐	ACUTE ☐
• Other				_____	Pedal ☐ ☐	
EARS					YES NO COMMENTS	CHRONIC ☐
• Responds to normal					Pacemaker	
voice tone					Peripheral Edema	Post Operative ☐
• Drainage					Chest Pain	
SPEECH					Jugular Vein	Other ☐
• Clear					Distention	
• Slurred					Extremity	_____
• Hoarse / raspy					Discoloration	_____
• Aphasic					Rt. Arm/Hand	
RESPIRATORY					Lt. Arm/Hand	
RESPIRATIONS				☐ Airway clearance,	Rt. Leg/Foot	
• Rate				ineffective	Lt. Leg/Foot	
• Labored				☐ Breathing pattern	GENITOURINARY	
BREATH SOUNDS				ineffective	VOIDING	☐ Urinary
• Clear				☐ Gas exchange;	• Normal	Elimination,
• Wheezes				impaired	• Frequency	alterations in
• Rales / Rhonchi				☐ IF PROBLEM	• Burning	pattern
				IDENTIFIED SEND		
COUGH				RESPIRATORY	Decreased Force of	
• Present				CONSULT	urinary stream	☐ Urinary
• Sputum				☐ Other	INCONTINENCE:	Retention
				_____	• Stress	
					• Nocturia	☐ Incontinence,
MUSCLE / SKELETAL						Total
EXTREMITIES				☐ Self Care deficit	UROSTOMY	
• Moves all on				☐ Mobility impaired,	DIALYSIS	
command				physical	If Yes: Hemo	☐ Incontinence,
WEAKNESS (specify)				☐ Activity intolerance	Peritoneal	Stress
RA___ LA___				comfort, alterations in	Routine schedule	
RL.___ LL.___				ACUTE ☐	Date of last Dialysis	☐ Comfort,
• Edema				CHRONIC ☐	Catheter insertion	alterations in
• Normal ambulation				☐ Tissue perfusion;	Date	
• Prosthesis (specify)				alterations in	Date of last	ACUTE ☐
			27053183.F10 02/12/99		menstrual period	CHRONIC ☐

(continues)

Figure 2-1 *(continued)*

sources and include family members, laboratory and diagnostic tests, other health care providers, and medical records.

Types of Data

Two types of information are collected through assessment: subjective and objective. **Subjective data** (symptoms) are information from the client's (sometimes family's) point of view and include feelings, perceptions, and concerns. The primary method

GASTROINTESTINAL				PROBLEM	INTEGUMENTARY	YES	NO	COMMENT	PROBLEM
ABDOMEN	YES	NO	COMMENT	Bowel	SKIN				☐ Other: _____
• Soft				elimination	• Color Normal				
• Distended				alterations in	• Warm, dry				☐ Tissue perfusion,
• Tenderness				☐ Diarrhea	• Turgor good				alterations in
ELIMINATION				☐ Constipation	• Bruises			☐ Referral to	☐ Skin integrity
• Bowel Sounds				☐ Incontinence,	abrasions,			Social Service	impairment of:
• Diarrhea				☐ Comfort	lacerations			(screen for	actual
• Constipation				altered pain	Color, Size,			neglect / abuse)	
• Incontinence				ACUTE ☐	Location				
• Ostomy				CHRONIC ☐					
Last B.M. Date:					• Poor hygiene				

SAFETY ASSESSMENT		
☐ (5) Age greater than 60	MEDICATIONS	
☐ (5) History of previous falls	☐ (5) Diuretics	
☐ (3) From nursing home	☐ (5) Laxatives / G.I. preps	
☐ (3) Has had sitter / companion	☐ (3) Antihypertensives	
at home	☐ (3) Antiseizures	
STATUS: MENTAL/PHYSICAL	☐ (5) Sedative / hypnotics	
☐ (5) Confused / Judgement Impaired	☐ (3) Analgesics	
☐ (5) Sensory impairment	☐ (3) Antipsychotics /	
☐ (5) Combative/Aggressive	antidepressants	
☐ (5) "Sundowners" Syndrome		
☐ (5) Noncompliance/uncooperativeness		
☐ (5) Paralysis / amputee	☐ LEVEL 1 (0-17)	
☐ (5) Weakness / debilitation	☐ LEVEL 2 (18-24)	
☐ (5) Urgent/frequent elimination needs	☐ LEVEL 3 (25 or greater)	
_____ TOTAL		
☐ Safety precautions implemented	☐ Patient/family instructed	
☐ Restraints per protocol	☐ Color coded band on	

Integumentary (right column continued):
• Rash, lesions — ☐ Skin integrity impairment of: potential
• Scars
• Dressing
• Pressure points intact — ☐ Tissue integrity, comfort, alterations in pain
  • coccyx
  • heels
  • elbows — ACUTE ☐
  • hips
  • ankles — CHRONIC ☐
  • cast edges
• Other _____ — WOUND CARE ☐
_____
E-Z graph
• Vascular access

Type _____ Insertion Date: _____
Site: _____ Purpose _____

NUTRITIONAL SCREENING
Indicate as appropriate for patient   Previous diet _____
☐ (8) TPN/Parental Nutrition
☐ (8) Tube Feeding
☐ (2) Unplanned weight loss or gain > 20 lbs in 3 months
☐ Referral to S.S. screen for neglect/abuse?
☐ (1) Loss of appetite/Eats less than 50% of meal
☐ (1) Nausea, vomiting or diarrhea
☐ (1) Difficulty chewing
☐ (1) Difficulty swallowing
*Diagnosis of:
☐ (2) Heart disease, hypertension, CHF, gestational diabetic, hepatic or renal failure, diabetic, anemia, cancer other than ENT, geriatric surgery
☐ (5) AIDS, malnutrition, DKA, decubitus ulcer, septic condition requiring ICU, burn patient, ENT cancer
☐ (1) modified diet; NPO for 48 hrs.
☐ (1) age > 65 years
*LAB VALUES: Albumin   Glucose   Hgb
☐ (1) 2.5 - 3.0   ☐ (1) <60 or   ☐ (1) male < 13
☐ (2) < 2.5   > 300   ☐ (1) female < 11
_____ TOTAL SCORE   ☐ SEND NUTRITION SCREEN
High Risk - 8 pts or >   CONSULT WITH TOTAL SCORE
Moderate Risk - 5-7 pts   OF 5 OR ABOVE AND IDENTIFY
Low Risk - 0-4 pts   SCORE OF PATIENT IN ORDER

SKIN BREAKDOWN POTENTIAL CHECKLIST
_____ (1) Fair: Major underlying disease, controlled
_____ (2) Poor: Uncontrolled underlying disease
MENTAL STATUS
_____ (1) Lethargic: Listless
_____ (2) Confused: Inappropriate communication
_____ (4) Comatose: Unresponsive
MOBILITY / ACTIVITY
_____ (2) Minor Deficit: Some limitation in movement
_____ (4) Major Deficit: Movement requires assistance
_____ (6) Immobile: No voluntary movement
INCONTINENCE
_____ (1) Mild: Stress incontinence, 1 BM / day
_____ (4) Frequent: No bladder control, BMs > 2-4 /day
_____ (6) Total: No bladder control, frequent / continuous BM
NUTRITION
_____ (2) Fair: Intake < body requirements, eats 75% or less
_____ (3) Poor: Eats 50% or less, started on TPN or tube feeding
_____ (4) Compromised: No intake, dehydrated
SKIN INTEGRITY
_____ (2) Fair: Single stage I or II
_____ (4) Poor: More than one break in skin integrity
_____ TOTAL SCORE OF 8 OR ABOVE, ENTER SKIN INTEGRITY POTENTIAL ON
PCP PROBLEM LIST, INITIATE PREVENTATIVE ADL's

PATIENT / SIGNIFICANT OTHER PARTICIPATION IN ADMISSION PROCESS			
1. Answered question Yes _____	No _____	3. Family/significant other present Yes _____	No _____
2. Volunteered information Yes _____	No _____	4. Plan of care reviewed with: Patient _____ Family / Significant other _____

5. Comments: 2705318-4.F10

Figure 2-1 *(continued)*

of collecting subjective data (also called symptoms) is the interview. The **health history**, a review of the client's functional health patterns prior to the current contact with the health care system, provides much of the subjective data.

Objective data (signs) are observable and measurable information that is obtained through both standard assessment techniques (Figure 2-2) and the results of laboratory and diagnostic testing. Table 2-1 provides examples of both subjective and objective data.

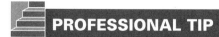

PROFESSIONAL TIP

Clients Who Were Adopted

Keep in mind that clients who were adopted will have varying degrees of knowledge about their biologic parents. Sensitivity to this issue is critical in gaining client trust during the interview process.

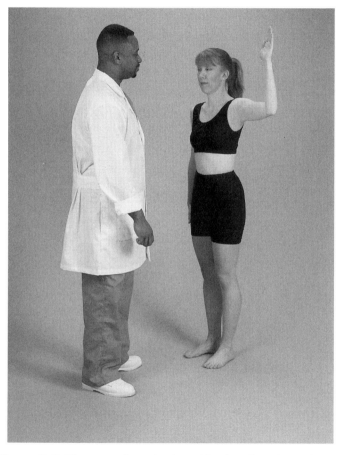

Figure 2-2 The nurse is gathering objective data through assessment of the client's ability to perform range-of-motion (ROM) activity.

Table 2-1 TYPES OF DATA

DATA

An African-American male, age 79, comes to the emergency room because he cannot move his left arm. The client states "It happened about an hour ago when my headache got worse. Now I am nauseated and dizzy."

The nurse takes his vital signs: T 99, P 100, R 28, BP 168/96, and observes that he cannot move his left arm and his face is flushed.

TYPE OF DATA

Subjective	Objective
headache	T 99, P 100
nausea	R 28, BP 168/96
dizziness	cannot move left arm
	flushed face

VALIDATING THE DATA

Objective data may add to or validate subjective data. A critical step in data collection, validation prevents omissions, misunderstandings, and incorrect inferences and conclusions (Figure 2-3). This process is particularly important if data sources are considered unreliable. For example, if a client is confused or unable to communicate, or if two sources provide conflicting data, it is necessary to seek further information or clarification. Findings should also be compared with normal values. Any grossly abnormal findings should be rechecked and confirmed.

ORGANIZING THE DATA

Collected data must be organized so as to be useful to the health care professional collecting the data and to others involved in the client's care. After being organized into categories, the data are clustered into groups of related pieces. **Data**

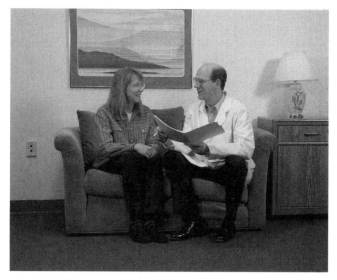

Figure 2-3 This nurse is validating information collected from the client during assessment.

clustering is the process of putting data together in order to identify areas of the client's problems and strengths. Many health care agencies use an admission assessment format, which assists the nurse in collecting and organizing data.

An **assessment model** is a framework that provides a systematic method for organizing data. A few of the many assessment models available to nurses are described following.

Hierarchy of Needs

Maslow's hierarchy of needs proposes that an individual's basic needs (physiologic) must be met before higher-level needs can be met. Use of a hierarchy of needs model requires initial assessment of all physiologic needs followed by assessment of higher-level needs.

Body Systems Model

The body systems model organizes data collection according to organ and tissue function in the various body systems (e.g., cardiovascular, respiratory, gastrointestinal). This method is sometimes referred to as the "medical model," because it is frequently used by physicians to investigate the presence or absence of disease.

Functional Health Patterns

Gordon's Functional Health Patterns (Gordon, 2000) provides a systematic framework for data collection that focuses on 11 functional health patterns. These functional health pattern areas allow the gathering and clustering of information about a client's usual patterns and any recent changes in order to ascertain whether the client's response is functional or dysfunctional. For example, the activity–exercise pattern is assessed for a client who recently experienced a stroke. Data collection would be focused on mobility and exercise patterns prior to the stroke, current muscle strength and joint mobility, and the effect of any changes on the client's lifestyle and functional ability. The 11 patterns are as follows:

- Health perception/health management pattern
- Nutritional/metabolic pattern
- Elimination pattern
- Activity/exercise pattern
- Cognitive/perceptual pattern
- Sleep/rest pattern
- Self-perception/self-concept pattern
- Role/relationship pattern
- Sexuality/reproductive pattern
- Coping/stress-tolerance pattern
- Value/belief pattern (Gordon, 2000)

Theory of Self-Care

The theory of self-care, developed by Orem (1995), is based on a client's ability to perform self-care activities. Self-care is learned behavior and deliberate action in response to need. It includes activities that an individual performs to maintain health. A major focus of this theory is the appraisal of the client's ability to meet self-care needs and the identification of existing self-care deficits. Because this theory focuses on deficits in care, it primarily addresses illness states. The self-care requisites are as follows:

- Maintenance of a sufficient intake of air
- Maintenance of a sufficient intake of water
- Maintenance of a sufficient intake of food
- Provision of care associated with elimination processes and excrements

- Maintenance of a balance between activity and rest
- Maintenance of a balance between solitude and social interaction
- Prevention of hazards to human life, human functioning, and human well-being
- Promotion of human functioning and development within social groups in accord with human potential, known human limitations, and the human desire to be normal (Orem, 1995)

INTERPRETING THE DATA

After data have been collected, the nurse can begin to develop impressions or inferences about the meaning of the data. Organizing data in clusters helps the nurse to recognize patterns of response or behavior. When data are placed in clusters, the nurse can:

- Distinguish between relevant and irrelevant data,
- Determine whether and where there are gaps in the data, and
- Identify patterns of cause and effect.

DOCUMENTING THE DATA

Assessment data must be recorded and reported. The nurse must make a judgment about which data are to be immediately reported to the head nurse and/or physician and which data need only be recorded at that time. Data that reflect a significant deviation from the normal (for example, rapid heart rate with irregular rhythm, severe difficulty in breathing, or a high level of anxiety) would need to be reported as well as recorded. Examples of data that need only to be recorded at the time include a report that prescribed medication has relieved a headache and a determination that an abdominal dressing is dry and intact.

Accurate and complete recording of assessment data is essential for communicating information to other health care team members. *Documentation is the basis for determining quality of care and should include appropriate data to support identified problems.*

SUMMARY

- The nurse uses the process of assessment to establish a database about the client, to form an interpersonal relationship with the client, and to provide the client with an opportunity to discuss health care concerns.
- The primary source of data is the client and is collected by both interview techniques and physical examination.
- Secondary sources of data include family members, laboratory and diagnostic tests, other health care providers, and medical records.
- Subjective data (also called symptoms) are the client's perceptions, concerns and feelings.
- Objective data (also called signs) are observable and measurable data obtained during physical examination and the results of laboratory and diagnostic tests.
- Documentation is the basis for determining quality of care and should include appropriate data to support identified problems.

Review Questions

1. Mrs. Rose was admitted to your unit 2 hours ago. The following data are recorded on her chart. Which data are objective?
   a. nausea
   b. headache
   c. pain in abdomen
   d. temperature 102°F

2. The following data are recorded on a client's admission assessment. Which of the data are subjective?
   a. nausea
   b. BP 120/80
   c. scars on abdomen
   d. redness on lower arms

3. The type of assessment most likely to be used in labor and delivery is:
   a. ongoing.
   b. focused.
   c. initial.
   d. comprehensive.

4. An assessment model often used to organize data is:
  a. data clustering.
  b. theory of health care.
  c. Maslow's hierarchy of needs.
  d. validation of systems model.

Critical Thinking Questions

1. How are comprehensive, focused, and ongoing assessments different?

2. Differentiate between subjective and objective data. Which are more important?

 WEB FLASH!

- Check the Internet for more information on Orem's theory of self-care and Gordon's functional health patterns.

References/Suggested Readings

Alfaro-LeFevre, R. (1998). *Applying nursing process* (4th ed.). Philadelphia: Lippincott Williams & Wilkins.

Alfaro-LeFevre, R. (1999). *Critical thinking in nursing: A practical approach* (2nd ed.). Philadelphia: W. B. Saunders Company.

American Nurses Association. (1991). *Standards of nursing practice.* Kansas City, MO: Author.

Bevis, E. O. (1989). *Curriculum building in nursing: A process* (3rd ed., Publication No. 15-2277). New York: National League for Nursing.

Edelman, C. L., & Mandle, C. L. (2001). *Health promotion throughout the lifespan* (5th ed.). St. Louis, MO: Mosby.

Gardner, P. (2002). *Nursing process.* Albany, NY: Delmar.

Gordon, M. (2000). *Manual of nursing diagnoses* (9th ed.). St. Louis, MO: Mosby.

Gregory, K. (2000). Nurse the patient! *RN, 63*(9), 52–54.

Heery, K. (2000). Straight talk about the patient interview. *Nursing2000, 30*(6), 66–67.

Humphrey, C. J. (1998). *Home care nursing* (3rd ed.). Gaithersburg, MD: Aspen.

Iyer, P. W., & Camp, N. H. (1999). *Nursing documentation: A nursing process approach*. St. Louis, MO: Mosby.

Johnson, D. (1959). A philosophy for nursing diagnosis. *Nursing Outlook, 7*, 198–200.

National Federation of Licensed Practical Nurses (NFLPN). (1996). *Nursing practice standards for the licensed practical/vocational nurse*. Garner, NC: Author.

North American Nursing Diagnosis Association (NANDA). (2001). *Nursing diagnoses: Definitions & classifications 2001–2002*. Philadelphia: Author.

Orem, D. E., Taylor, S. G., & Renpenning, K. (2001). *Nursing: Concepts of practice* (6th ed.). St. Louis, MO: Mosby.

Paul, R. W. (1995). *Critical thinking: How to prepare students for a rapidly changing world*. Santa Rosa, CA: Foundation for Critical Thinking.

Seaback, W. (2001). *Nursing process: Concepts & application*. Albany, NY: Delmar

White, L. (2001). *Foundations of nursing: Caring for the whole person*. Albany, NY: Delmar.

White, L. (2002). *Basic nursing: Foundations of skills & concepts*. Albany, NY: Delmar.

Wiedenbach, E. (1963). The helping art of nursing. *AJN, 63*(11), 54–57.

Wilkinson, J. M. (2001). *Nursing process and critical thinking* (3rd ed.). Englewood Cliffs, NJ: Prentice Hall.

Yoder Wise, P. S. (1998). *Leading and managing in nursing* (2nd ed.). St. Louis, MO: Mosby.

CHAPTER 3

DIAGNOSIS

Upon completion of this chapter, you should be able to:
- *Define key terms.*
- *Differentiate between nursing diagnosis and medical diagnosis.*
- *Write nursing diagnosis statements in both the two-part statement and three-part statement.*
- *Compare the three types of nursing diagnosis: actual, risk, and wellness.*

KEY TERMS

actual nursing diagnosis	nursing diagnosis
analysis	potential complication
collaborative problem	risk nursing diagnosis
defining characteristics	synthesis
etiology	wellness nursing diagnosis
medical diagnosis	

INTRODUCTION

Diagnosis, the second step in the nursing process, involves further **analysis** (breaking down the whole into parts that can be examined) and **synthesis** (putting data together in a new way) of the data that have been collected. Formulation of the list of nursing diagnoses is the outcome of this process. According to NANDA, a **nursing diagnosis**:

is a clinical judgment about individual, family, or community responses to actual or potential health problems/life processes. A nursing diagnosis provides the basis for selection of nursing interventions to achieve outcomes for which the nurse is accountable. (NANDA, 2001)

The nursing diagnoses developed during this phase of the nursing process provide the basis for client care delivered through the remaining steps.

Clients receive both medical and nursing diagnoses. Table 3-1 compares the two categories of diagnoses. It is important to have a clear understanding of the nature of a nursing diagnosis as compared to a **medical diagnosis** (clinical judgment by the physician that identifies or determines a specific disease, condition, or pathologic state). Table 3-2 compares selected nursing and medical diagnoses.

Table 3-1 COMPARISON OF NURSING AND MEDICAL DIAGNOSIS	
NURSING DIAGNOSIS	**MEDICAL DIAGNOSIS**
Recognizes situations that the nurse is licensed and qualified to treat.	Recognizes conditions the physician is licensed and qualified to treat.
Concentrates on the client's responses to actual or risk health problems or life processes.	Concentrates on illness, injury, or disease processes.
Varies as the client's responses and/or health problems change.	Stays the same until a cure is realized or client dies.
EXAMPLE:	EXAMPLE:
Nausea	Cholelithiasis
Acute Pain	
	Surgery
Acute Pain	Cholecystectomy
Impaired Physical Mobility	

Table 3-2 COMPARISON OF SELECT NURSING AND MEDICAL DIAGNOSES	
NURSING DIAGNOSES	**MEDICAL DIAGNOSES**
Decreased Cardiac Output	Congestive heart failure
Ineffective Breathing Pattern	
Risk for Imbalanced Fluid Volume	
Impaired Physical Mobility	Meniere's disease
Death Anxiety	Lung cancer
Ineffective Airway Clearance	Chronic obstructive pulmonary disease
Ineffective Breathing Pattern	
Anxiety	

The nurse uses critical-thinking and decision-making skills in developing nursing diagnoses. This process is facilitated by asking questions such as:

- Are there problems here?
- If so, what are the specific problems?
- What are some possible causes of the problems?
- Is there a situation involving risk factors?
- What are the risk factors?
- Can a problem develop if preventive measures are not taken?
- If so, under what circumstances?
- Has the client indicated a desire for a higher level of wellness in a particular area of function?
- What are the client's strengths?
- What cultural factors, values, or beliefs are involved for this client?
- What data are available to answer these questions?
- Are more data needed to answer the question?
- If so, what are some possible sources of the data that are needed?

COMPONENTS OF A NURSING DIAGNOSIS

Several formats have been used to structure nursing diagnosis statements. Two formats that are frequently seen in the nursing literature are the two-part statement and the three-part statement. The two-part statement is NANDA approved and is used by most nurses mainly because of its brief and precise format. The three-part statement is usually required of nursing students and is preferred by those nurses desiring to strengthen the diagnostic statement by including specific manifestations. Refer to Appendix A for a list of NANDA-approved nursing diagnoses.

Two-Part Statement

The first component, the actual nursing diagnosis, is a problem statement or diagnostic label that describes the client's response to an actual or potential health problem or a wellness condition.

The second component of a two-part nursing diagnosis statement is the etiology. The **etiology** is the related cause or contributor to the problem and is identified in the complete NANDA diagnosis description. The diagnostic label and etiology are linked by the term *related to* (R/T). Because the NANDA list of nursing diagnoses is constantly evolving, there may be times when no etiology is provided. In such cases, the nurse should attempt to describe likely contributing factors to the client's condition. Examples of a two-part nursing diagnosis statement are *Feeding Self-care Deficit* R/T perceptual/cognitive impairment and *Delayed Growth and Development* R/T separation from significant others.

Three-Part Statement

The nursing diagnosis can also be expressed as a three-part statement. As in the two-part statement, the first two components are the diagnostic label and the etiology. The third component consists of **defining characteristics** (collected data, also known as signs and symptoms, subjective and objective data, or clinical manifestations). The third part is joined to the first two components with the connecting phrase *as evidenced by* (AEB). An example of a three-part nursing diagnosis statement is *Impaired Gas Exchange* R/T ventilation perfusion imbalance AEB respiratory rate of 40.

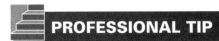

PROFESSIONAL TIP

Benefits of Nursing Diagnosis

- Nursing diagnosis is unique in that it focuses on a client's *response* to a health problem rather than on the problem itself, and it provides a structure through which nursing care can be delivered.
- Nursing diagnosis provides a means for effective communication.
- Holistic client, family, and community-focused care are facilitated with the use of nursing diagnosis

WRITING THE NURSING DIAGNOSIS STATEMENT

The nursing diagnosis selected from the NANDA list becomes the diagnostic label, the first part of the diagnosis statement. Etiologies are also chosen from the NANDA descriptions. The appropriate etiology is selected and joined to the first part of the statement with the "related to" phrase. Table 3-3 compares selected NANDA-approved diagnoses in two- and three-part formats.

TYPES OF NURSING DIAGNOSES

Analysis of the collected data leads the nurse to make a nursing diagnosis. NANDA identifies three types of nursing diagnoses. They are:

- An **actual nursing diagnosis** indicates that a problem exists; it is composed of the diagnostic label, related factors, and signs and symptoms. An example of an actual diagnosis is *Situational Low Self-esteem* R/T loss (first chair trumpet in band) AEB self-negating verbalizations "I'm no good anymore."
- A **risk nursing diagnosis** (potential problem) indicates that a problem does not yet exist, but that special risk factors are present. A risk diagnosis is composed of the phrase *Risk for* followed by the diagnostic label and a list of the specific risk factors. An example of a risk diagnosis is *Risk for Situational*

Table 3-3 EXAMPLES OF NURSING DIAGNOSES WRITTEN AS TWO- AND THREE-PART STATEMENTS

TWO-PART STATEMENT	THREE-PART STATEMENT
Toileting Self-care Deficit R/T neuro-muscular impairment	*Toileting Self-care Deficit* R/T neuromuscular impairment AEB paralysis of right side of body
Impaired Swallowing R/T mechanical obstruction	*Impaired Swallowing* R/T/ mechanical obstruction AEB tracheostomy tube
Impaired Urinary Elimination R/T urinary tract infection	*Impaired Urinary Elimination* R/T urinary tract infection AEB frequency and dysuria
Impaired Memory R/T fluid and electrolyte imbalance	*Impaired Memory* R/T fluid and electrolyte imbalance AEB inability to recall recent or past events
Impaired Home Maintenance R/T individual/family member disease or injury	*Impaired Home Maintenance* individual/family member disease or injury AEB repeated lice infestations

PROFESSIONAL TIP

Nursing Diagnosis

• The nursing diagnosis must be developed from the data, never the other way around.

• Do not try to fit a client to a nursing diagnosis; rather, select the appropriate diagnosis from the data cues presented by the client. Failure to do so may result in errors in developing a nursing diagnosis.

Low Self-esteem R/T unrealistic self-expectations AEB receiving "B" in two college courses while working full-time (expected "A").

- A **wellness nursing diagnosis** indicates the client's expression of a desire to attain a higher level of wellness in some area of function. For example, a wife who has been caring for her husband who had a stroke two months ago asks the nurse about meeting with other wives who are/have been in a similar situation. The nurse would make a wellness diagnosis of *Readiness for Enhanced Family Coping*.

Examples of the three types of diagnoses are shown in Table 3-4.

After formulation, the nursing diagnoses should be discussed with the client, if possible. If this is not possible, the diagnoses may be discussed with family members. Finally, the list of nursing diagnoses is recorded on the client's record. After this list has been developed and recorded, the remainder of the client's care plan can be completed. The list of nursing diagnoses is not static. It is dynamic, changing as more data are collected and as client goals and client responses to interventions are evaluated.

Table 3-4 TYPES OF NURSING DIAGNOSES

TYPE	EXAMPLE
Actual Diagnosis	*Perceived Constipation* R/T faulty appraisal AEB expectation of passage of stool at same time every day
Risk Diagnosis	*Risk for Aspiration* R/T decreased cough and gag reflexes
Wellness Diagnosis	*Readiness for Enhanced Spiritual Well-being*

COLLABORATIVE PROBLEMS

Carpenito (2000) discusses situations in which nurses intervene in collaboration with other disciplines. She defines **collaborative problems** as "certain physiologic complications that nurses monitor to detect onset or changes in status. Nurses manage collaborative problems using physician-prescribed and nursing-prescribed interventions to minimize the complications of the events." She has identified 52 specific collaborative problems grouped under 9 generic problem categories. For example under the generic collaborative problem category of *Potential Complication* (PC): *Respiratory* are the specific collaborative problems of "PC: Hypoxemia, PC: Atelectasis/pneumonia, PC: Tracheobronchial Constriction, and PC: Pneumothorax."

The collaborative problem statement *always* begins with **Potential Complication** or PC. This differentiates the collaborative problem statement from a nursing diagnosis. A benefit of using collaborative problem statements is that they identify, and thus keep the nurses aware of, the potential complications a client may encounter. As in the example above, the specific potential complication for a client with a respiratory problem would be listed on the care plan.

SUMMARY

• Diagnosis, the second step in the nursing process, involves further analysis and synthesis of the data and results in a list of nursing diagnoses.

• Nursing diagnoses contribute to a clearer conceptualization of knowledge unique to nursing, improved communication among nurses and other health care professionals, and promotion of individualized client care.

• The types of nursing diagnoses are actual, risk, and wellness.

• Nursing diagnoses deal with client responses to actual or potential health problems/life processes while medical diagnoses identify or determine a specific disease, condition, or pathologic state.

Review Questions

1. A nursing diagnosis is a clinical judgment:
   a. about a pathologic state.
   b. identifying a specific disease or condition.
   c. about a client's responses to health problems.
   d. determining a client's responses to life processes.

2. The first component of a nursing diagnosis statement is:
   a. etiology.
   b. synthesis.
   c. diagnostic label.
   d. defining characteristics.

3. The second component of a nursing diagnosis statement is:
   a. etiology.
   b. assessment of data.
   c. diagnostic label.
   d. defining characteristics.

4. A wellness diagnosis indicates the client:
   a. has no health problems.
   b. just wants to get well.
   c. is only at risk for a health problem.
   d. desires to attain a higher level of wellness.

Critical Thinking Questions

1. How are a nursing diagnosis and a medical diagnosis different?

2. Differentiate between the three types of nursing diagnoses: actual, risk, and wellness.

WEB FLASH!

- Check out NANDA's Web site, www.nanda.org. What information do you find? How is this helpful to client care?

References/Suggested Readings

Alfaro-LeFevre, R. (1998). *Applying nursing process* (4th ed.). Philadelphia: Lippincott Williams & Wilkins.

Alfaro-LeFevre, R. (1999). *Critical thinking in nursing: A practical approach* (2nd ed.). Philadelphia: W. B. Saunders Company.

American Nurses Association. (1991). *Standards of nursing practice*. Kansas City, MO: Author.

Carpenito, L. J. (2000). *Nursing diagnosis: Application to clinical practice* (8th ed.). Philadelphia: Lippincott Williams & Wilkins.

Edelman, C. L., & Mandle, C. L. (2001). *Health promotion throughout the lifespan* (5th ed.). St. Louis, MO: Mosby.

Gardner, P. (2002). *Nursing process.* Albany, NY: Delmar.

Gordon, M. (2000). *Manual of nursing diagnoses* (9th ed.). St. Louis, MO: Mosby.

Iyer, P. W., & Camp, N. H. (1999). *Nursing documentation: A nursing process approach.* St. Louis, MO: Mosby.

National Federation of Licensed Practical Nurses (NFLPN). (1996). *Nursing practice standards for the licensed practical/vocational nurse.* Garner, NC: Author.

North American Nursing Diagnosis Association (NANDA). (2001). *Nursing diagnoses: Definitions & classifications 2001–2002.* Philadelphia: Author.

Orem, D. E., Taylor, S. G., & Renpenning, K. (2001). *Nursing: Concepts of practice* (6th ed.). St. Louis, MO: Mosby.

Seaback, W. (2001). *Nursing process: Concepts & application.* Albany, NY: Delmar.

White, L. (2001). *Foundations of nursing: Caring for the whole person.* Albany, NY: Delmar.

White, L. (2002). *Basic nursing: Foundations of skills & concepts.* Albany, NY: Delmar.

Wilkinson, J. M. (2000). *Nursing diagnosis handbook with NIC interventions and NOC outcomes.* Englewood Cliffs, NJ: Prentice Hall.

Wilkinson, J. M. (2001). *Nursing process and critical thinking* (3rd ed.). Englewood Cliffs, NJ: Prentice Hall.

CHAPTER 4

PLANNING AND OUTCOME IDENTIFICATION

Upon completion of this chapter, you should be able to:
- *Define key terms.*
- *Differentiate between initial, ongoing, and discharge planning.*
- *Describe how to prioritize nursing diagnoses.*
- *Discuss how goals are established.*

KEY TERMS

dependent nursing intervention	interdependent nursing intervention
discharge planning	long-term goal
expected outcome	nursing care plan
goal	nursing intervention
independent nursing intervention	ongoing planning
initial planning	planning
	short-term goal

INTRODUCTION

Planning combines with outcome identification to comprise the third step of the nursing process and includes both the formulation of guidelines that establish the proposed course of nursing action in the resolution of nursing diagnoses and the development of the client's plan of care. After the nursing diagnoses have been developed and the client's strengths have been identified, planning can begin.

PLANNING

The planning of nursing care occurs in three phases: initial, ongoing, and discharge. Each type of planning contributes to the coordination of the client's comprehensive plan of care. **Initial planning** involves development of a preliminary plan of care by the nurse who performs the admission assessment and gathers the comprehensive admission assessment data. Because of progressively shorter lengths of hospitalization, initial planning is important in addressing each problem and in correlating nursing care to hasten resolution of these problems. **Ongoing planning** entails continuous updating of the client's plan of care. As new information about the client is gathered and evaluated, revisions may be generated and the initial plan of care further individualized to the client. **Discharge planning** involves critical anticipation and preparing for the client's needs after discharge.

The planning phase involves several tasks:

- Prioritizing the list of nursing diagnoses
- Identifying and writing client-centered long- and short-term goals and outcomes (outcome identification)
- Developing specific nursing interventions
- Recording the entire nursing care plan in the client's record

PRIORITIZING THE NURSING DIAGNOSES

Prioritizing the nursing diagnoses involves making decisions about which diagnoses are the most important and therefore require attention first. One of the most common methods of selecting priorities is to consider Maslow's hierarchy of needs, which leads the nurse to consider a life-threatening diagnosis more urgent than a non-life-threatening diagnosis. After basic physiologic needs (e.g., respiration, nutrition, temperature, hydration, and elimination) are met to some degree, the nurse would then consider needs on the next level of the hierarchy (e.g., safe environment, stable living condition, affection, and self-worth) and so on up the hierarchy until all the client's nursing diagnoses have been prioritized.

Alfaro-LeFevre (1999) suggests a three level approach to prioritizing client problems (nursing diagnoses).

- **First-level priority problems (immediate):**
  Airway problems
  Breathing problems
  Cardiac/circulation problems
  Signs (vital signs)

- **Second-level priority problems (immediate, after treatment for first level problems is initiated):**
  Mental status change
  Acute pain
  Acute urinary elimination problems
  Untreated medical problems requiring immediate attention (e.g., a diabetic who has not had insulin)
  Abnormal lab values
  Risks of infection, safety, or security (for client or others)

- **Third-level priority problems:**
  Health problems that do not fit in the first and second level categories

She also proposes that *sometimes* the priority order may change. For example, if acute pain causes breathing problems, managing the pain may have the higher priority; if abnormal lab values are life-threatening, then they have a higher priority. Table 4-1 illustrates the prioritizing process.

IDENTIFYING OUTCOMES

Outcome identification includes establishing goals and expected outcomes, which together provide guidelines for individualized nursing interventions and establish evaluation criteria to measure the effectiveness of the nursing care plan.

Goals

A **goal** is an aim, intent, or end. Goals are broad statements that describe the intended or desired change in the client's condition or behavior. Client-centered goals are established in collaboration with the client whenever possible. Goal statements refer to the diagnostic label (or problem statement) of the nursing diagnosis. If the client or significant others are unable to participate in goal development, the nurse assumes that responsibility until the client is able to participate. Client-centered goals ensure that nursing care is individualized and focused on the client.

Table 4-1 PRIORITIZING NURSING DIAGNOSES

NURSING DIAGNOSIS	PRIORITIZING METHOD	PRIORITY
Decreased Cardiac Output R/T altered heart rate rhythm	Maslow, physiologic Alfaro-LeFevre, cardiac/circulatory	High High
Diarrhea R/T travel	Maslow, physiologic	High
	Alfaro-LeFevre, untreated medical problem	Moderate
Relocation Stress Syndrome R/T isolation from family/friends	Maslow, safety and security Alfaro-LeFevre, risk to security	Moderate Moderate
Disturbed Sleep Pattern R/T daytime activity pattern	Maslow, safety and security Alfaro-LeFevre, other health problems	Moderate Low
Ineffective Coping R/T inadequate resources available	Maslow, self-esteem Alfaro-LeFevre, other health problems	Low Low

A **short-term goal** is an objective statement that outlines the desired resolution of the nursing diagnosis over a short period of time, usually a few hours or days (less than a week). Short-term goals focus on the etiology component of the nursing diagnosis. A **long-term goal** is an objective statement that outlines the desired resolution of the nursing diagnosis over a longer period of time, usually weeks or months. Long-term goals focus on the problem component of the nursing diagnosis. Table 4-2 provides examples of short-term and long-term goals.

Expected Outcomes

After the goals have been established, the expected outcomes can be identified based on those goals. An **expected outcome** is a detailed, specific statement that describes the

Table 4-2 SHORT- AND LONG-TERM GOALS

NURSING DIAGNOSIS: *DISTURBED BODY IMAGE* R/T SURGERY FOR BREAST CANCER

Short-term Goals (focus on etiology)	Long-term Goals (focus on problem)
Will verbalize loss of breast	Will verbalize acceptance of change in physical self
Will identify negative feelings about body	
Will touch chest where breast was	

methods through which the goal will be achieved and includes aspects such as direct nursing care, client teaching, and continuity of care. Outcomes must be measurable, time-limited, and realistic. Several expected outcomes may be required for each goal (Table 4-3). After goals and expected outcomes have been established, nursing interventions are formulated to enable the client to reach the goals.

DEVELOPING SPECIFIC NURSING INTERVENTIONS

A **nursing intervention** is an action performed by the nurse that helps the client achieve the results specified by the goals and expected outcomes. Nursing interventions refer directly to the related factors in the actual or wellness nursing diagnoses and to the risk factors in risk nursing diagnoses. If the nursing interventions can remove or reduce the related factors and the risk factors, the problem can be resolved or prevented.

For each nursing diagnosis, there may be a number of nursing interventions. Nursing interventions are individualized and are stated in specific terms. Examples of nursing interventions are as follows:

- Assist client to turn, cough, and deep breathe q 2 h beginning at 0800, 2/10
- Teach nipple care when breastfeeding at 1000, 2/11
- Weigh client at each visit

Table 4-3 GOAL AND EXPECTED OUTCOMES

NURSING DIAGNOSIS: *IMPAIRED URINARY ELIMINATION* R/T URINARY TRACT INFECTION AEB FREQUENT URINATION IN SMALL AMOUNTS

Goal	Expected Outcomes
Client will have improved urinary elimination.	Client will take antibiotic as ordered.
	By next visit, client will identify three factors to prevent a urinary tract infection.
	In 2 days, client will have a plan to increase water intake.
	By next visit, client will be urinating at least 150 mL at 2 hour or longer intervals.

NURSING DIAGNOSIS: *POWERLESSNESS* R/T ILLNESS-RELATED REGIMEN AEB NONPARTICIPATION IN CARE OR DECISION MAKING WHEN OPPORTUNITIES ARE PROVIDED

Goal	Expected Outcomes
Client will participate in care and decision making.	In 2 days, client will participate in one aspect of own care each day.
	Client will state preference in decision-making situation within 1 week.

After interventions have been formulated for each diagnosis, they are recorded on the client's care plan. As is true with other steps in the nursing process, the list of interventions is not static. As the nurse interacts with the client, assesses responses to interventions, and evaluates those responses, interventions may change.

CATEGORIES OF NURSING INTERVENTIONS

Nursing interventions are classified into one of three categories: independent, interdependent, or dependent. **Independent nursing interventions** are nursing actions that are initiated by the nurse and do not require direction or an order from another health care professional. In many states, the nursing practice act allows independent nursing interventions with regard to activities such as daily living, health education, health promotion, and counseling. An example of an independent nursing intervention is the nurse's elevating a client's edematous extremity.

Interdependent nursing interventions are those actions that are implemented in a collaborative manner by the nurse in conjunction with other health care professionals. A client care conference with an interdisciplinary health care team results in interdependent nursing interventions. For example, the nurse may assist a client to perform an exercise taught by the physical therapist.

Dependent nursing interventions are those actions that require an order from a physician or another health care professional. An example of a dependent intervention is administration of a medication. Although this intervention requires specific nursing knowledge and responsibilities, it is not within the realm of legal practice for licensed practical/vocational nurses (LP/VNs) or registered nurses (RNs) unless they are advance practice registered nurses working in certain states, to prescribe medications. When administering medications, the nurse is responsible for knowing the classification, pharmacologic action, normal dosage, adverse effects, contraindications, and nursing implications of the drug. Therefore, dependent nursing interventions, like all nursing actions, must be guided by appropriate knowledge and judgment.

RECORDING THE NURSING CARE PLAN

The **nursing care plan** is a written guide that organizes data about a client's care into a formal statement of the strategies that will be implemented to help the client achieve optimal health.

Nursing care plans usually include components such as assessment, nursing diagnoses, goals and expected outcomes, nursing interventions, and evaluation. The nurse begins the nursing care plan on the day of admission and continually updates and individualizes the client's plan of care until discharge.

There are several types of care plans including student-oriented, standardized, institutional, and computerized care plans. The student-oriented care plan promotes learning of problem-solving skills, the nursing process, verbal and written communication skills, and organizational skills. This comprehensive care plan offers great depth for teaching the process of planning care and usually includes a scientific rationale for each intervention. Although educational programs vary, the student-oriented care plan usually begins with assessment and proceeds in a sequential manner until it concludes with the evaluation of the care plan.

The standardized care plan is a preplanned, preprinted guide for the nursing care of client groups with common needs. This type of care plan generally follows the nursing process format. The nurse may use standardized care plans when a client has predictable, commonly occurring problems. Individualization may be accomplished by the inclusion of additional handwritten notes regarding unusual problems.

Institutional nursing care plans are concise documents that become a part of the client's medical record after discharge. The Kardex nursing care plan is an example of this type of care plan and is frequently used. The institutional nursing care plan may simply include the nursing diagnoses, nursing interventions, and evaluation. In addition, the Kardex nursing care plan may be expanded to include assessment, nursing diagnoses, goals, implementation, and evaluation. Figure 4-1 provides an example of an institutional care plan.

Computers are used for creating and storing nursing care plans and can generate both standardized and individualized nursing care plans. The nurse selects appropriate diagnoses from a menu suggested by the computer, which then lists possible goals and nursing interventions. The nurse has the option of reading the client's plan of care from the computer screen or printing an updated working copy. Figure 4-2 is an example of a computerized nursing care plan.

Nursing Diagnosis	Nursing Interventions	Evaluation
Ineffective Breastfeeding R/T deficient knowledge AEB inability to latch on to the maternal breast correctly	*1. Teach various breastfeeding positions and techniques to encourage the infant. 2. Stay with mother during feeding and assist as needed.*	*1. Client tried the various positions and techniques. 2. Client able to assist infant to latch on to breast correctly.*
Risk for Constipation R/T abdominal muscle weakness and hemorrhoids	*1. Assess daily for bowel movement frequency and consistency. 2. Encourage more fluid and fiber intake.*	*1. Bowel movement daily, very firm consistency. 2. Asking for fruit between meals; drinking 8 oz water every 2 hours when awake.*

Figure 4-1 Handwritten Institutional Care Plan

SUMMARY

- Planning and outcome identification, the third step in the nursing process, involves prioritizing nursing diagnoses, identifying and writing client-centered goals and client outcomes, developing nursing interventions, and recording the plan of care in the client's record.
- The client's plan of care, also called the nursing care plan, documents health care needs, coordinates nursing care, promotes continuity of care, encourages communication among health care team members, and promotes quality nursing care.
- When prioritizing nursing diagnoses, Maslow's hierarchy of needs or Alfaro-LeFevre's three levels of priority are common methods to use.
- Outcome identification provides guidelines for individualized nursing interventions and establishes evaluation criteria to measure effectiveness of the nursing care plan.

Client Name: Jane White   **Sex:** Female

Age: 77   **Temp:** 101.5   **BP:** 168/74   **Pulse:** 124 O_2 **Sat:** 89%

Client Health History

Ms. White has smoked two to three packs of cigarettes a day for the past 60 years. She was diagnosed with COPD 4 years ago and has required supplemental oxygen at 2 L/min for the past 18 months. Her chief complaints are increasing dyspnea on exertion and a cough, which is sometimes productive, yielding thick, green-yellow sputum. She states, "I don't know why I'm coughing up this awful stuff."

Assessment Findings

Respiratory Rate 38

Sonorous and sibilant wheezes on expiration in the posterior lung fields with superimposed coarse crackles heard in the right posterior lower lung field.

Unable to ambulate to the bathroom or complete other ADLs because of dyspnea

Nursing Diagnosis: *Ineffective Breathing Pattern* R/T diseased lungs, infection, and increased secretions AEB severe dyspnea, elevated blood pressure, and increased pulse

Goals: Ms. White will:

1. Have a normal respiratory rate.

2. Have clear lung sounds.

3. Be able to complete ADLs.

4. Increase oral fluid intake

Planning and Intervention

Intervention	Rationale
1. Assist client in assuming a high Fowler's position	Maximizes thoracic cavity space, decreases pressure from diaphragm and abdominal organs, facilitates use of accessory muscles

(continues)

Figure 4-2 Computer-Generated Nursing Care Plan (Format from Delmar's *Electronic Care Plan Maker,* by S. Sheehy, 1998, Albany, NY: Delmar. Content from *Medical-Surgical Nursing: An Integrated Approach* (2nd ed.) by L. White and G. Duncan, 2002, Albany, NY: Delmar. Copyright 2002 by Delmar)

2. Provide humidified, low flow (2 L/min) oxygen, as ordered — Provides some supplemental oxygen to improve oxygenation and makes secretions less viscous

3. Administer bronchodilators, as ordered — Reduces bronchospasm and improves air flow

4. Administer IV fluids and increase oral fluids (2000–3000 mL/day as tolerated), as ordered — Improves hydration, decreases secretions

5. Administer expectorants, as ordered — Decreases secretions of previously ineffective cough

6. Administer antibiotics, as ordered — Eradicates respiratory infection or pneumonia and reduces secretions and end inflammation

7. Administer xanthines (aminophylline, theophylline), as ordered — Decreases smooth muscle spasm and edema of the mucosa

8. Administer non-narcotic cough suppressants, as ordered — Coughing can lead to fatigue. It is important for COPD clients to get adequate rest and not become fatigued

Evaluation/Outcome

Client's breathing returns to a more normal pattern

Client is able to cough up secretions

Client is able to ambulate to bathroom and complete ADLs

Client is drinking at least 2000 mL/day of water

Nursing Diagnosis: *Impaired Gas Exchange* R/T lower airway (alveolar) wall destruction preventing adequate exchange of gases of respiration and airway obstruction (secretions) preventing adequate oxygenation AEB severe dyspnea, tachypnea, elevated blood pressure, increased pulse, and decreased oxygen saturation

Goals: Ms. White will:

1. Have O_2 saturation of 95%.

2. Have normal vital signs.

(continues)

Figure 4-2 *(continued)*

Planning and Interventions

Intervention	Rationale
1. Assist client in assuming a high Fowler's position	Decreases the work of breathing (at least through crisis period)
2. Administer medications to loosen secretions, as ordered	Decreases secretions of previously ineffective cough
3. Provide humidified, low flow (2 L/min) oxygen, as ordered	Improves oxygenation, moistens thick secretions

Evaluation/Outcome

Client will exhibit improved O_2 saturation

Client will exhibit normal vital signs

Figure 4-2 *(continued)*

Review Questions

1. The client's plan of care includes:
   a. collected documentation of all team members providing care for the client.
   b. physician orders, demographic data, and medication administration and rationales.
   c. client's nursing diagnoses, goals, expected outcomes, and the nursing interventions.
   d. client assessment data, medical treatment regimen and rationales, and diagnostic test results and significance.

2. When establishing priorities for a client's plan of nursing care, the nurse should rank life-threatening diagnoses as the highest priorities and which as the lowest priorities?
   a. safety-related needs
   b. client needs regarding referral agencies
   c. the client's social, love, and belonging needs
   d. needs of family members and friends who are involved in plan of care

3. The essential components of an expected outcome are:
   a. nursing diagnosis, interventions, and expected client behavior.
   b. target date, nursing action, measurement criteria, and desired client behavior.

    c. nursing client behavior, target date, and conditions under which the behavior occurs.

    d. client behavior, measurement criteria, conditions under which the behavior occurs, and target date.

4. The nursing care plan:

    a. may be handwritten or computer generated.

    b. is never changed once it has been worked out.

    c. always includes all aspects of the nursing process.

    d. is not part of the client's record and is discarded when client is discharged.

Critical Thinking Questions

1. Why is it important to prioritize nursing diagnoses?

2. Differentiate between the three categories of nursing interventions: independent, interdependent, and dependent.

3. How are goals and outcomes different?

WEB FLASH!

• What resources are available on the internet for planning and outcome identification?

References/Suggested Readings

Alfaro-LeFevre, R. (1998). *Applying nursing process* (4th ed.). Philadelphia: Lippincott Williams & Wilkins.

Alfaro-LeFevre, R. (1999). *Critical thinking in nursing: A practical approach* (2nd ed.). Philadelphia: W. B. Saunders Company.

American Nurses Association. (1991). *Standards of nursing practice.* Kansas City, MO: Author.

Bevis, E. O. (1989). *Curriculum building in nursing: A process* (3rd ed., Publication No. 15-2277). New York: National League for Nursing.

Carpenito, L. J. (2000). *Nursing diagnosis: Application to clinical practice* (8th ed.). Philadelphia: Lippincott Williams & Wilkins.

DeLaune, S., & Ladner, P. (2002). *Fundamentals of nursing: Standards & practice* (2nd ed.). Albany, NY: Delmar.

Edelman, C. L., & Mandle, C. L. (2001). *Health promotion throughout the lifespan* (5th ed.). St. Louis, MO: Mosby.

Gardner, P. (2002). *Nursing process*. Albany, NY: Delmar.

Gordon, M. (1998, September 30). Nursing nomenclature and classification system developing. *On-line Journal of Issues in Nursing* [Online]. Available: http://www.nursingworld.org

Humphrey, C. J. (1998). *Home care nursing* (3rd ed.). Gaithersburg, MD: Aspen.

Iyer, P. W., & Camp, N. H. (1999). *Nursing documentation: A nursing process approach*. St. Louis, MO: Mosby.

National Federation of Licensed Practical Nurses (NFLPN). (1996). *Nursing practice standards for the licensed practical/vocational nurse*. Garner, NC: Author.

North American Nursing Diagnosis Association (NANDA). (2001). *Nursing diagnoses: Definitions & classifications 2001–2002*. Philadelphia: Author.

Oermann, M., & Huber, D. (1999). Patient outcomes: A measure of nursing's value. *AJN, 99*(9), 40–47.

Orem, D. E., Taylor, S. G., & Renpenning, K. (2001). *Nursing: Concepts of practice* (6th ed.). St. Louis, MO: Mosby.

Paul, R. W. (1995). *Critical thinking: How to prepare students for a rapidly changing world*. Santa Rosa, CA: Foundation for Critical Thinking.

Seaback, W. (2001). *Nursing process: Concepts & application*. Albany, NY: Delmar.

Tucker, S., Canobbio, M., Paquette, E., & Wills, M. (2000). *Patient care standards: Collaborative planning & nursing interventions* (7th ed.). St. Louis, MO: Mosby.

White, L. (2001). *Foundations of nursing: Caring for the whole person*. Albany, NY: Delmar.

White, L. (2002). *Basic nursing: Foundations of skills & concepts*. Albany, NY: Delmar.

Wilkinson, J. M. (2001). *Nursing process and critical thinking* (3rd ed.). Englewood Cliffs, NJ: Prentice Hall.

Yoder Wise, P. S. (1998). *Leading and managing in nursing* (2nd ed.). St. Louis, MO: Mosby.

CHAPTER 5

IMPLEMENTATION

LEARNING OBJECTIVES

Upon completion of this chapter, you should be able to:
- *Define key terms.*
- *Discuss the types of skills that nurses must possess in order to perform the nursing interventions.*
- *Differentiate between specific order, standing order, and protocol.*
- *Describe what is to be documented and/or reported regarding nursing interventions.*

KEY TERMS

assign	protocol
delegation	specific order
implementation	standing order

INTRODUCTION

The fourth step in the nursing process is implementation. **Implementation** involves the execution of the nursing care plan derived during the planning phase. It consists of performing nursing activities (interventions) that have been planned to meet the goals set with the client. It also involves the **delegation** (process of transferring a select nursing task to a licensed individual who is competent to perform that specific task) of some nursing interventions to staff members or **assigning** a specific nursing task to assistive (unlicensed) personnel capable of competently performing the task. The nurse remains accountable for appropriate delegation and supervision of care provided by unlicensed individuals.

REQUIREMENTS FOR EFFECTIVE IMPLEMENTATION

Implementation involves many skills. The nurse must continue to assess the client's condition before, during, and after each nursing intervention. Assessment prior to intervention implementation provides the nurse with baseline data. Assessment during and after intervention implementation allows the nurse to detect positive or negative responses the client may have to the intervention. If negative responses occur during the intervention, the nurse must take appropriate action. If positive responses occur, the nurse adds this information to the database for use in evaluating the efficacy of the intervention.

The nurse must also possess psychomotor skills, interpersonal skills, and cognitive skills to perform the nursing interventions that have been planned. The nurse uses psychomotor skills to safely and effectively perform nursing activities. Nurses must be able to both handle medical equipment with a high degree of competency and perform such skills as giving injections, changing dressings, and helping the client perform range-of-motion (ROM) exercises.

Interpersonal skills are necessary as the nurse interacts with the client and the family to collect data, provide information in teaching sessions, and offer support in times of anxiety. The nurse–client relationship is established and maintained through the use of therapeutic communication. Interaction between and among members of the health care team promotes collaboration and enhances the holistic care of the client.

Cognitive skills enable the nurse to make appropriate observations, understand the rationale for the activities performed, ask the appropriate questions, and make decisions about those things that need to be done. Critical thinking is an important element within the cognitive domain because it helps the nurse analyze data, organize observations, and apply prior knowledge and experiences to current client situations.

It is important for the nurse to be familiar with the agency's procedure and policy manuals. Most procedures can have variations in how they are performed and still be effective, efficient, and safe. The procedure manual delineates how a particular agency expects procedures to be performed. The policy manual explains the agency's expected method of handling various situations.

TYPES OF NURSING INTERVENTIONS

Nursing interventions are written as orders in the care plan and may be nurse initiated, physician initiated, or derived from collaboration with other health care professionals. Interventions can be implemented on the basis of specific orders, standing orders, or protocols.

A **specific order** is an order written in a client's medical record or nursing care plan by a physician or nurse especially for that individual client; it is not used for any other client.

A **standing order** is a standardized intervention written, approved, and signed by a physician that is kept on file within health care agencies to be used in predictable situations or in circumstances requiring immediate attention. Nurses can implement standing orders in these situations after assessing the client and identifying the primary or emerging problem. An example of a physician-initiated standing order on an inpatient unit would be specification of certain medications to be administered for a common headache.

A **protocol** is a series of standing orders or procedures that should be followed under certain specific conditions. The protocol defines those interventions that are permissible and those circumstances under which the nurse is allowed to implement the measures. Health care agencies or individual physicians frequently have standing orders or protocols for client preparation for diagnostic tests or for immediate interventions in life-threatening circumstances. These protocols prevent needless duplication of effort with regard to writing the same orders

 COMMUNITY/HOME HEALTH CARE

Standing Orders

Nurses in home health care agencies may have standing orders for administering certain medications or ordering laboratory tests when indicated.

repeatedly for different clients, often saving valuable time in critical situations.

DOCUMENTING AND REPORTING INTERVENTIONS

The implementation step also involves documentation and reporting. Data to be recorded include the client's condition prior to the intervention, the specific intervention performed, the client's response to the intervention, and client outcomes. This documentation not only constitutes a legal record, but also allows for valuable communication among other health care team members for purposes of ensuring continuity of care and evaluating progress toward expected outcomes. In addition, written documentation provides data necessary for reimbursement for services.

Verbal interaction among health care providers is also essential for communicating current information about clients. Communication between nurses generally occurs at the change of shift, when the responsibility for care changes from one nurse to another. Nursing students must communicate relevant information to the nurse responsible for their clients when they leave the unit. Information that should be shared in the verbal report includes:

• Those activities completed and those yet to be completed,
• Status of current relevant problems,
• Any abnormalities or changes in assessment,
• Results of treatments,
• Diagnostic tests scheduled or completed (and results if known), and
• Newly identified problems (last 8 hours).

All communication—both written and verbal—must be objective, descriptive, and complete. All communication must include observations rather than opinions and be stated or written to convey an accurate picture of the client's condition. Thorough and detailed communication of implementation activities is fundamental to ensuring that client care and progress toward goals can be adequately evaluated.

Reporting will be covered in more detail in Chapter 12.

SUMMARY

- The implementation step of the nursing process is directed toward meeting client needs, resulting in health promotion, prevention of illness, illness management, or health restoration.
- Interventions can be nurse initiated, physician initiated, or collaborative in origin.
- Implementation involves assessment skills, psychomotor skills, interpersonal skills, and cognitive skills.
- Interventions may be implemented on the basis of specific orders, standing orders, or protocols.
- Documentation of interventions provides valuable communication among health care team members to ensure continuity of care and evaluation of client progress toward expected outcomes.

Review Questions

1. Implementation involves the nurse performing nursing interventions and sometimes:
   a. writing protocols.
   b. delegating some interventions.
   c. seeking reimbursement for services.
   d. eliminating the need for critical thinking.

2. For effective implementation, the nurse must possess assessment skills, interpersonal skills, psychomotor skills and also:
   a. cognitive skills.
   b. deductive skills.
   c. communication skills.
   d. eye-hand coordination skills.

3. Documentation of nursing interventions:
   a. provides jobs for transcribers.
   b. ensures progress toward expected outcomes.
   c. constitutes a legal record of care to the client.
   d. frees nurses from performing complete assessments.

Critical Thinking Questions

1. Why are the six items listed at the end of the chapter for the nursing student to report before leaving the unit important? What are the implications if this information is not reported?

2. Differentiate between specific orders, standing orders, and protocols.

WEB FLASH!

- Can you find specific sites or resources dealing with the nursing process?
- What resources are available on the internet for nurses needing assistance with the nursing process?

References/Suggested Readings

Alfaro-LeFevre, R. (1998). *Applying nursing process* (4th ed.). Philadelphia: Lippincott Williams & Wilkins.

Alfaro-LeFevre, R. (1999). *Critical thinking in nursing: A practical approach* (2nd ed.). Philadelphia: W. B. Saunders Company.

American Nurses Association. (1991). *Standards of nursing practice.* Kansas City, MO: Author.

Edelman, C. L., & Mandle, C. L. (2001). *Health promotion throughout the lifespan* (5th ed.). St. Louis, MO: Mosby.

Gardner, P. (2002). *Nursing process.* Albany, NY: Delmar.

Humphrey, C. J. (1998). *Home care nursing* (3rd ed.). Gaithersburg, MD: Aspen.

Iyer, P. W., & Camp, N. H. (1999). *Nursing documentation: A nursing process approach.* St. Louis, MO: Mosby.

National Federation of Licensed Practical Nurses (NFLPN). (1996). *Nursing practice standards for the licensed practical/vocational nurse.* Garner, NC: Author.

North American Nursing Diagnosis Association (NANDA). (2001). *Nursing diagnoses: Definitions & classifications 2001–2002.* Philadelphia: Author.

Orem, D. E., Taylor, S. G., & Renpenning, K. (2001). *Nursing: Concepts of practice* (6th ed.). St. Louis, MO: Mosby.

Seaback, W. (2001). *Nursing process: Concepts & application*. Albany, NY: Delmar.

Tucker, S., Canobbio, M., Paquette, E., & Wills, M. (2000). *Patient care standards: Collaborative planning & nursing interventions* (7th ed.). St. Louis, MO: Mosby.

White, L. (2001). *Foundations of nursing: Caring for the whole person*. Albany, NY: Delmar.

White, L. (2002). *Basic nursing: Foundations of skills & concepts*. Albany, NY: Delmar.

Wilkinson, J. M. (2001). *Nursing process and critical thinking* (3rd ed.). Englewood Cliffs, NJ: Prentice Hall.

Yoder Wise, P. S. (1998). *Leading and managing in nursing* (2nd ed.). St. Louis, MO: Mosby.

CHAPTER 6

EVALUATION

LEARNING OBJECTIVES

Upon completion of this chapter, you should be able to:
- *Define key terms.*
- *Identify the components of the nursing process affected by evaluation.*
- *Document evaluation of client care on the client's record.*
- *Discuss how nursing audits are performed.*

KEY TERMS

evaluation   nursing audit

INTRODUCTION

Once care is provided to a client, it is appropriate to check if the care was of value to the client in meeting the established goals. This process is called evaluation.

EVALUATION

Evaluation, the fifth step in the nursing process, involves determining whether the client goals have been met, partially met, or not met. If a goal has been met, the nurse must then decide whether nursing activities should cease or continue in order for status to be maintained. If a goal has been partially met or not met, the nurse must reassess the situation. Data are collected to determine both the reasons the goal has not been achieved and the necessary modifications to the plan of care.

Among a number of possible reasons that goals are not met or are only partially met are the following:

- The initial assessment data were incomplete.
- The nursing diagnoses were inappropriate.
- The goals and expected outcomes were not realistic.
- The time frame was too optimistic.
- The goals and/or the nursing interventions planned were not appropriate for the client or situation.
- Implementation of the plan was not fully carried out.

Evaluation is a fluid process that is dependent on all the other components of the nursing process. As shown in Figure 6-1, evaluation affects, and is affected by, assessment, diagnosis, planning and outcome identification, and implementation of nursing care. Table 6-1 shows the way evaluation is woven into every phase of the nursing process. Ongoing evaluation is essential if the nursing process is to be implemented appropriately. As Alfaro-LeFevre (1998) states:

> When we evaluate early, checking whether our information is accurate, complete, and up-to-date, we're able to make corrections *early*. We avoid making decisions based on

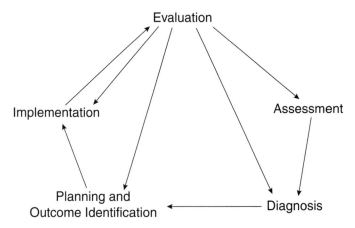

Figure 6-1 Relationship of Evaluation to the Other Components of the Nursing Process: Evaluation Impacts Every Component

Table 6-1 INTERACTION BETWEEN THE OTHER COMPONENTS OF THE NURSING PROCESS AND EVALUATION

NURSING PHASE COMPONENTS	EVALUATION QUESTIONS
Assessment	Are data relevant to client needs? Are data obtained by appropriate methods? Are data collected from multiple, varied sources? Is a systematic, organized method used in collecting data? Is data collection thorough and complete?
Diagnosis	Are diagnoses based on the collected data? Is each nursing diagnosis complete? Are nursing diagnoses client centered and relevant? Are nursing diagnoses comprehensive? Are nursing diagnoses used to guide planning and implementation of care?
Planning and Outcome Identification	Are nursing diagnoses prioritized? Are expected outcomes relevant to nursing diagnoses? Are outcomes realistic and achievable? Are resources (including team members) used efficiently? Are care plans documented? Is care plan revised according to the client's needs?

(continues)

Table 6-1 INTERACTION BETWEEN THE OTHER COMPONENTS OF THE NURSING PROCESS AND EVALUATION *continued*	
NURSING PHASE COMPONENTS	**EVALUATION QUESTIONS**
Implementation	Is plan of care followed by all team members? Are necessary resources available? Do nursing actions assist client in meeting expected outcomes? Are client expected outcomes achieved? Does documentation reflect the client's status, including responses to nursing interventions?

outdated, inaccurate, or incomplete information. Early evaluation enhances our ability to act safely and effectively. It improves our *efficiency* by helping us stay focused on priorities and avoid wasting time continuing useless actions.

NURSING AUDIT

A **nursing audit** is a method of evaluating the quality of care provided to clients. A nursing audit can focus on implementation of the nursing process, on client outcomes, or on both in order to evaluate the quality of care provided. The nursing audit is a follow-up evaluation that not only evaluates the quality of care of an individual client but also provides an evaluation of overall care given in that health care facility. During a nursing audit the evaluators look for documentation of all five components of the nursing process in the client records.

Health care facilities each have an ongoing nursing audit committee to evaluate the quality of care given. The nursing

COMMUNITY/HOME HEALTH CARE

Effectiveness of Care

When evaluating the effectiveness of care, the home health care nurse can use the following questions to examine client achievement of expected outcomes:

• Were the goals realistic in terms of client abilities and time frame?
• Were there external variables (for example, housing problems, impaired family dynamics) that prevented goal achievement?
• Did the family have the resources (for example, transportation) to assist in meeting the goals?
• Was the care coordinated with other providers to facilitate efficient delivery of care?

audit committee reviews client records after discharge of the clients. They examine the records for data related to:

• Safety measures,
• Treatment interventions and client responses to those interventions,
• Preestablished outcomes used as a basis for interventions,
• Discharge planning,
• Client teaching, and
• Adequacy of staffing patterns.

SUMMARY

• Evaluation, the fifth step in the nursing process, measures the effectiveness of nursing interventions by the examination of the goals and expected outcomes, which provide direction for the plan of care and serve as standards against which the client's progress is measured.
• Nursing audit serves to evaluate how the nursing process was followed in caring for clients, based on the documentation in the client's record.

CASE STUDY

Mr. Jona is a client on your unit. A 70-year-old widower, he was admitted 2 days ago with a broken left hip. While bowling with his church league, Mr. Jona tripped, fell, fractured his hip, and sprained his right wrist. He recently retired from an administrative position with a large company and moved to Florida from his home in Iowa. He has two children: one son who lives in Shumak, Washington, and a daughter who lives in Ono, New York. Mr. Jona lives alone in a one-bedroom apartment approximately 10 blocks from the hospital. In 4 days, Mr. Jona will be discharged and referred to the home health division for follow-up care.

The following questions will guide your development of a nursing care plan for the case study.

1. What assessments must be done with regard to Mr. Jona's going home?
2. Which three nursing diagnoses may apply to Mr. Jona?
3. What goals and outcomes may be appropriate for Mr. Jona?
4. What nursing interventions may be appropriate to meet the goals?
5. What evaluation questions should be asked?

Review Questions

1. Evaluation should take place:
   a. at the end of each shift.
   b. after the client has gone home.
   c. during each aspect of the nursing process.
   d. only after implementation of the nursing care plan.

2. A nursing audit:
   a. focuses on nursing interventions.
   b. evaluates the quality of client care.
   c. is performed on each unit at the end of each shift.
   d. comes under the auditing division of the health care agency.

Critical Thinking Questions

1. When and how should evaluation be accomplished?

2. Why is evaluation necessary?

3. Why are nursing audits important?

 WEB FLASH!

- Check the Internet for information related to evaluation as applied to the nursing process.

References/Suggested Readings

Alfaro-LeFevre, R. (1998). *Applying nursing process* (4th ed.). Philadelphia: Lippincott Williams & Wilkins.

Alfaro-LeFevre, R. (1999). *Critical thinking in nursing: A practical approach* (2nd ed.). Philadelphia: W. B. Saunders Company.

American Nurses Association. (1991). *Standards of nursing practice.* Kansas City, MO: Author.

Edelman, C. L., & Mandle, C. L. (2001). *Health promotion throughout the lifespan* (5th ed.). St. Louis, MO: Mosby.

Gardner, P. (2002). *Nursing process.* Albany, NY: Delmar.

Humphrey, C. J. (1998). *Home care nursing* (3rd ed.). Gaithersburg, MD: Aspen.

Iyer, P. W., & Camp, N. H. (1999). *Nursing documentation: A nursing process approach.* St. Louis, MO: Mosby.

National Federation of Licensed Practical Nurses (NFLPN). (1996). *Nursing practice standards for the licensed practical/vocational nurse.* Garner, NC: Author.

Orem, D. E., Taylor, S. G., & Renpenning, K. (2001). *Nursing: Concepts of practice* (6th ed.). St. Louis, MO: Mosby.

Seaback, W. (2001). *Nursing process: Concepts & application.* Albany, NY: Delmar.

White, L. (2001). *Foundations of nursing: Caring for the whole person.* Albany, NY: Delmar.

White, L. (2002). *Basic nursing: Foundations of skills & concepts.* Albany, NY: Delmar.

Wilkinson, J. M. (2001). *Nursing process and critical thinking* (3rd ed.). Englewood Cliffs, NJ: Prentice Hall.

Yoder Wise, P. S. (1998). *Leading and managing in nursing* (2nd ed.). St. Louis, MO: Mosby.

UNIT
2

Documentation

CHAPTER 7

DOCUMENTATION AS COMMUNICATION

LEARNING OBJECTIVES

Upon completion of this chapter, you should be able to:
- *Define key terms.*
- *Explain the five purposes of documentation in health care.*
- *Identify the various sheets in a client's medical record.*

KEY TERMS

advance directive
documentation

informed consent

INTRODUCTION

Communication is a dynamic, continuous, and multidimensional process for sharing information as determined by standards or policies. Reporting and recording are the major communication techniques used by health care providers in directing client-based decision making and continuity of care. The medical record serves as a legal document for recording all client activities initiated by all health care practitioners.

DOCUMENTATION DEFINED

Documentation is defined as written evidence of:

- The interactions between and among health professionals, clients, their families, and health care organizations;

- The administration of tests, procedures, treatments, and client education; and
- The results of, or client's response to, diagnostic tests and interventions (Eggland & Heinemann, 1994).

Documentation provides written records that reflect client care provided on the basis of assessment data and the client's response to interventions.

In implementing the nursing process, nurses rely on the documentation tools of client charts and other documents that facilitate a logical sequencing of events. All the tools used by nurses to record their nursing care should form a system. Systematic documentation is critical because it presents the care administered by nurses in a logical fashion, as follows:

- Assessment data, obtained through interview, observation, and physical examination, identify the client's specific alteration and lay the foundation for the nursing care plan.
- The identified alteration in functional health pattern directs the formulation of a nursing diagnosis.
- The nursing diagnoses trigger the client's expected outcomes (both short- and long-term goals) and accompanying supportive nursing interventions—the planning and implementation phases.
- The effectiveness of the nursing interventions in achieving the client's expected outcomes becomes the criterion for evaluation, determining the need for subsequent reassessment and revision of the plan of care (Eggland & Heinemann, 1994; Iyer & Camp, 1999).

The system becomes a vehicle for expressing each phase of the nursing process. Nurses rely on systems that provide thorough, accurate charting reflective of the nurse's decision-making ability and the client's plan of care. The nurse's critical-thinking skills, judgments, and evaluations must be clearly communicated through proper documentation.

PURPOSES OF HEALTH CARE DOCUMENTATION

Professional responsibility and accountability are two primary reasons for documentation. As the professional responsibility of all health care practitioners, documentation provides written evidence of the practitioner's accountability to the client, the institution, the profession, and society. Other reasons to document include communication, education, research, satisfaction of legal and practice standards, and reimbursement.

Communication

Documentation is a communication method that confirms the care provided to the client and clearly outlines all important information regarding the client. Thorough documentation provides:

- Accurate data needed to plan the client's care and to ensure continuity of care;
- A method of communication among the health care team members responsible for the client's care;
- Written evidence of those things done for the client, the client's response, and any revisions made in the plan of care;
- Evidence of compliance with professional practice standards (e.g., those of the American Nurses Association [ANA]);
- Evidence of compliance with accreditation criteria (e.g., those of the Joint Commission on Accreditation of Healthcare Organizations [JCAHO]);
- A resource for review, audit, reimbursement, education, and research; and
- A written legal record to protect the client, institution, and practitioner.

The client's medical record contains documents for record keeping. The type of documents that constitute the medical record in a given health care institution is determined by that institution. Table 7-1 outlines the content of the documents generally found in a client's medical record.

Education

The documentation contained in the client's medical record is used for the purpose of education. Health care students can use the medical record as a tool to learn about disease processes, complications, medical and nursing diagnoses, and interventions. The results from physical examinations and laboratory and diagnostic testing provide valuable information regarding specific diagnoses and interventions.

Nursing students can enhance their critical-thinking skills by examining the records in chronologic order, analyzing the results, and following the health care team's plan of care,

Table 7-1   DOCUMENTS OF THE CLIENT MEDICAL RECORD

DOCUMENT	INFORMATION
Face Sheet	*Demographic data:* name, client's identifying number, address, telephone number, date of birth, place of birth, sex, race, marital status, religion, name and address of closest relative, social security number, admission date and hour, type of admission
	Financial Data: expected payer(s), insured's name and sex, client relationship to insured, employer's name and location, group name, insurance group number, insured's policy number
	Clinical Data: admitting diagnosis, admitting diagnosis-related group (DRG), client's advance directive (if has one)
	Discharge Data (to be entered by the physician on discharge of client): name of attending physician, discharge date and hour, principal diagnosis and other diagnoses, external cause of injury code, procedures and dates, operating physician(s), disposition of client
Medical History and Physical Examination	Client's description of chief complaint, present and past illnesses, personal and family histories, and review of systems as elicited by the physician, findings of physician's assessment of all body systems
Nursing Admission Assessment	Data from interview and physical assessment performed by the nurse
Physician's Orders	Physician's written or verbal orders to admit, to direct client's diagnostic and therapeutic course, and to discharge

(continues)

Table 7-1 DOCUMENTS OF THE CLIENT MEDICAL RECORD *continued*

DOCUMENT	INFORMATION
Consultation Report	Findings of a physician whose opinion or advice is requested by another physician for evaluation and/or treatment of a client
Physician's Progress Notes	Provides a pertinent, chronologic report of the client's course in the hospital and reflects any change in condition and response to treatment. May also contain notes by other members of the health care team (e.g., dietary or social service)
Laboratory Reports	Results from laboratory tests ordered by the physician
Radiology Reports	Radiologists interpretation of radiologic and fluoroscopic diagnostic services
Nuclear Medicine	Describes diagnostic studies and therapeutic procedures performed using radiopharmaceutical agents
Graphic Sheet	Various client parameters, most commonly: T, P, R, and BP. May also include weight, diet, I&O
Client Care Plan (Nursing Plan of Care)	Treatment plan including nursing diagnoses or problem list, client goals, nursing actions, and evaluation
Nurses' Notes	Details care and treatments provided, client's response to care and treatments, achievement of expected outcomes that do not duplicate information on Flow Sheet (if used)
Flow Sheet	All routine interventions that can be indicated by a check mark or other simple descriptor

(continues)

Table 7-1 DOCUMENTS OF THE CLIENT MEDICAL RECORD *continued*

DOCUMENT	INFORMATION
Medication Administration	Contains all medications administered orally, topically, by injection, inhalation, and infusion in one place; includes date, time, dosage, route of administration, and name of professional administering the drug. Routine, PRN, and single dose orders generally have separate sections.
Consent Forms	*Admission:* gives the institution and physician permission to treat
	Surgical: explains the reason for and nature of the treatment, the risks, complications, alternate forms of treatment, no treatment, consequences of treatment or procedure. Sometimes surgical and anesthesia consents are separate so that responsibility is placed appropriately.
	Blood Transfusion: gives specific permission to administer blood or blood products
	Other: procedure specific consent forms, participate in research project, photography
Client Education Record	Describes the nurse's teaching to the client, family, or other caregiver and the learner's response
Health Care Team Record	Used by respiratory, physical therapy, dietary when physician's progress are used only by physicians
Nursing Discharge Summary	Contains brief summary of care provided, medications, teaching, and other instructions (e.g., return appointment, referrals), discharge status, and mode of discharge

(continues)

Table 7-1 DOCUMENTS OF THE CLIENT MEDICAL RECORD *continued*	
DOCUMENT	**INFORMATION**
Discharge Summary	Review of events describing the client's illness, investigation (diagnostic studies), treatment, response, and condition at discharge. Instructions to the client and plans for follow-up care are included.
Advance Directive	Both a living will and a durable power of attorney for health care are considered advance directives. Federal law requires that all clients be given written information about their rights so they can make decisions concerning medical care. An advance directive is not required to be in a client's medical record.
Other Documents	These may or may not be in a client's medical record: Operative report, Anesthesia report, Pathology report, Transfusion record, Rehabilitation report, Critical pathway, Restraint record, and Autopsy report.

including the way it was developed, implemented, and evaluated. Students and all health care professionals must be aware of confidentiality issues before reading any client's chart.

Research

Researchers rely heavily on the client's medical record as a clinical data source to determine whether clients meet the research criteria for a study. Documentation also can direct the need for research. For example, if documentation demonstrates an increased infection rate in association with intravenous catheters, researchers can identify and study the variables that may be associated with the increased infection rate.

Legal and Practice Standards

"Failure to document appropriately is a key factor in clinical mishaps and a pivotal issue in many malpractice cases" (Springhouse, 1999). *The client's medical record is a legal document, and in the case of a lawsuit, it is the record that serves as the description of exactly what happened to a client.* If it is not documented in the client's record, it did not occur. In 80% to 85% of malpractice lawsuits involving client care, the medical record is the determining factor in providing proof of significant events (Iyer & Camp, 1999). The legal issues of documentation require:

* Legible and neat writing,
* Correct spelling and grammar,
* Use of authorized abbreviations,
* Date and time for each entry, and
* Accurate, factual, time-sequenced, descriptive notations.

To focus attention on the importance of communicating and documenting all information, Fiesta (1991) cites *Ramsey v. Physician Memorial Hospital.* An emergency room nurse failed to communicate to the physician that the mother of two pediatric clients had found a tick on one of the two children. One of the children later died from Rocky Mountain spotted fever. The physician had questioned the health team about ticks because of the children's elevated temperature, but was told nothing. The court dismissed the hospital from liability, but the apellate court held the hospital liable because the nurse had failed to communicate to the physician the information obtained from the mother about the tick.

The nurse is responsible for documenting on the chart both that the physician was notified and the significant information that was orally communicated. If the physician does not respond in a way that indicates an understanding of the urgency of the information, the nurse must document the physician's response and notify the supervisor of the situation. Nurses are responsible for the care the client receives and can be held liable if appropriate interventions are not implemented in a timely manner when information is available that would dictate otherwise.

Informed Consent   **Informed consent** is a competent client's ability to make health care decisions based on full disclosure of

PROFESSIONAL TIP

The Importance of Communication

Important information obtained from an assessment and warranting immediate intervention should not only be documented in the medical record but also communicated orally to those other practitioners involved in the client's care. The element of time must direct decision making when critical information is obtained.

PROFESSIONAL TIP

Consent from Sedated Clients

Sedated clients should never be requested or allowed to sign an informed consent. Because the client may not be capable of understanding the nature of and risks associated with the procedure, the consent will be invalid, and the nurse and institution will be at legal risk. Instead, either wait for the client to be competent and free of sedation (usually 4 hours after administration of the last medication that alters the level of consciousness) or have a legally acceptable family member brought into the decision.

the benefits, risks, and potential consequences of a recommended treatment plan and of alternative treatments, including no treatment, and the client's voluntary agreement to the treatment. Informed consent can be given either orally or in writing. Written consent is not required by law; however, it does document the process of informed consent which could be crucial in the event of a lawsuit (Olson-Chavarriaga, 2000) (Figure 7-1).

Although the physician who is to perform the procedure is responsible for obtaining the client's informed consent, the nurse is often the person who actually has the client sign the form. The nurse's signature as a witness on an informed consent form is vouching that the client or the appropriate surrogate is the person signing and that the person signing understands that a consent form is being signed (Olson-Chavarriaga, 2000).

TO THE PATIENT: You have the right as a patient to be informed about your condition and the recommended surgical, medical, or diagnostic procedure to be used so that you may make the decision whether or not to undergo the procedure after knowing the risks and hazards involved. This disclosure is not meant to scare or alarm you, but is simply an effort to make you better informed so you may give or withhold your consent to the procedure. Any questions or concerns you may have with respect to the proposed procedure, its risks, complications, or benefits should be directed to your treating physician.

I (we) voluntarily request Dr. _____ as my physician, and such associates, technical assistants and other health care providers as they may deem necessary to treat my condition, which has been explained to me as: _____

I (we) understand that the following surgical, medical, and/or diagnostic procedures are planned for me, and I (we) voluntarily consent and authorize these procedures: _____

I (we) understand that my physician may discover other or different conditions which require additional or different procedures than those planned. I (we) authorize my physician, and such associates, technical assistants, and other health care providers, to perform such procedures which are advisable in their professional judgment.

I (we) [DO] [DO NOT] consent to the use of blood and blood products as deemed necessary.

I (we) understand that no warrant or guarantee has been made to me as a result or cure.

Just as there may be risks and hazards in continuing my present condition without treatment, there are also risks and hazards related to the performance of the surgical, medical, and/or diagnostic procedures planned for me. I (we) realize that common to surgical, medical, and/or diagnostic procedures is the potential for infection, blood clots in veins and lungs, hemorrhage, allergic reactions, and even death. I (we) realize that the following risks and hazards may occur in connection with this particular procedure:

I (we) understand that anesthesia involves additional risks and hazards, but I (we) request the use of anesthetics for the relief and protection from pain during the planned and additional procedures. I (we) realize the anesthesia may have to be changed, possibly without explanation to me (us).

I(we) understand that certain complications may result from the use of any anesthetic, including respiratory problems, drug reaction, paralysis, brain damage, or even death. Other risks and hazards which may result from the use of general anesthetics range from minor discomfort to injury to vocal cords, teeth, or eyes. I (we) understand that other risks and hazards resulting from spinal or epidural anesthetics include headache, chronic pain, remote possibility of nerve injury, hematoma, infection, septic and aseptic meningitis, nausea, vomiting, itching, and urinary retention.

I (we) consent to the photographing of the operations or procedures to be performed, including appropriate portions of the body, for medical, scientific, or educational purposes, provided my identity is not revealed by descriptive texts accompanying the picture.

I (we) consent to the disposition by hospital authorities of any tissues or parts which may be removed.

I (we) have been given the opportunity to ask questions about my conditions, alternative forms of anesthesia and treatment, risks of non-treatment, the procedures to be used, and the risks and hazards involved, and I (we) believe that I (we) have sufficient information to give this informed consent.

I (we) certify that I (we) have discussed the proposed procedures and risks with my physician; that this form has been fully explained to me; that I (we) have read it or have had it read to me (us); that the blank spaces have been filled in; and that I (we) understand its contents.

DATE: _____   TIME: _____

                                                                    A.M./P.M.

Patient/other legally responsible person   Witness Name
(Minor patient and parent/guardian signature)

SPOHN HEALTH SYSTEM
CORPUS CHRISTI, TEXAS 78404

DISCLOSURE AND CONSENT-
MEDICAL AND SURGICAL PROCEDURES
PATIENT CARE SERVICES

2704980   NEW: 05/82
                      REVISED: 05/96

Figure 7-1 Disclosure and Consent—Medical and Surgical Procedures (Courtesy CHRISTUS Spohn Health System, Corpus Christi, TX)

Advance Directives   An **advance directive** (i.e., living will [Figure 7-2] and durable power of attorney for health care [Figure 7-3]) is written instructions about an individual's health care preferences regarding life-sustaining measures that guide family members and health care professionals as to those treatment options that should or should not be considered in the event that the individual is unable to decide. This effectively

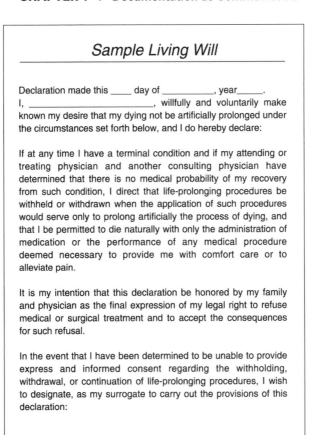

Sample Living Will

Declaration made this _____ day of _____, year_____.
I, _____, willfully and voluntarily make known my desire that my dying not be artificially prolonged under the circumstances set forth below, and I do hereby declare:

If at any time I have a terminal condition and if my attending or treating physician and another consulting physician have determined that there is no medical probability of my recovery from such condition, I direct that life-prolonging procedures be withheld or withdrawn when the application of such procedures would serve only to prolong artificially the process of dying, and that I be permitted to die naturally with only the administration of medication or the performance of any medical procedure deemed necessary to provide me with comfort care or to alleviate pain.

It is my intention that this declaration be honored by my family and physician as the final expression of my legal right to refuse medical or surgical treatment and to accept the consequences for such refusal.

In the event that I have been determined to be unable to provide express and informed consent regarding the withholding, withdrawal, or continuation of life-prolonging procedures, I wish to designate, as my surrogate to carry out the provisions of this declaration:

(continues)

Figure 7-2 Sample Living Will (Reprinted by permission of Choice in Dying, 200 Varick Street, New York, NY 10014)

allows clients, while competent, to participate in end-of-life decisions and to choose the types of life-sustaining procedures they wish to be performed.

State Nursing Practice Acts   In an attempt to recognize and control the practice of nursing, nursing practice acts, on a state-by-state basis, establish guidelines to ensure safe practice and to demonstrate accountability to society. *The standards of care, as set forth in the practice acts, are based on the phases of the nursing process and require compliance as evidenced in documentation.* Nurses should be familiar with the practice act of the state in which they work.

Name: _____
Address: _____
_____ Zip Code: _____
Phone: _____

I wish to designate the following person as my alternate surrogate, to carry out the provisions of this declaration should my surrogate be unwilling or unable to act on my behalf:

Name: _____
Address: _____
_____ Zip Code: _____
Phone: _____

Additional instructions (optional):

I understand the full importance of this declaration, and I am emotionally and mentally competant to make this declaration.
Signed: _____

Witness 1:
   Signed: _____
   Address: _____

Witness 2:
   Signed: _____
   Address: _____

Figure 7-2 *(continued)*

Joint Commission on Accreditation of Healthcare Organizations   The JCAHO surveys health care facilities to measure compliance with its standards for safe health care provision. Although facilities voluntarily submit to this accreditation process, reimbursement eligibility for Medicare, Medicaid, and private funding is dependent on JCAHO accreditation.

The JCAHO no longer requires that health care organizations have traditional nursing care plans, but documentation of an individualized plan of care must be evident for each client (JCAHO, 1998). The JCAHO's standards require:

• The involvement of the client or family in the development of the plan, which must be documented in the medical record, and

---

Part I. Durable Power of Attorney for Health Care

• If you do NOT wish to name an agent to make health care decisions for you, write your initials in the box

[Initials]

This form has been prepared to comply with the "Durable Power of Attorney for Health Care Act" of Missouri.

1. Selection of agent. I appoint:
Name:_____
Address:_____

It is suggested that only one Agent be named. However, if more than one Agent is named, anyone may act individually unless you specify otherwise.

Telephone:_____
as my Agent.

2. Alternate Agents. Only an Agent named by me may act under this Durable Power of Attorney. If my Agent resigns or is not able or available to make health care decisions for me, or if an Agent named by me is divorced from me or is my spouse and legally separated from me, I appoint the person(s) named below (in the order named if more than one):

First Alternate Agent	Second Alternate Agent
Name:_____	Name:_____
Address:_____	Address:_____
Telephone:_____	Telephone:_____

This is a Durable Power of Attorney, and the authority of my Agent shall not terminate if I become disabled or incapacitated.

(continues)

Figure 7-3 Durable Power of Attorney for Health Care and Health Care Directive (Reprinted with permission of the Missouri Bar)

- Interdisciplinary planning and implementation of all aspects of care.

The use of interdisciplinary tools has proved an effective approach to documenting client and family education for agencies not yet using critical pathways. By complying with JCAHO's client and family teaching standards, one medical center, through the use of an interdisciplinary record, increased its education documentation rate from 30% to 84% (Tucker, 1995).

During the accreditation survey (or process), the reviewer looks for evidence of an organized and systematic method of monitoring and evaluating client care as reflected through documentation in the medical record. Documenting the steps of the nursing process ensures compliance with JCAHO's plan of care requirements.

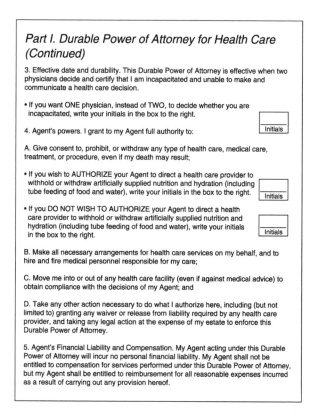

Part I. Durable Power of Attorney for Health Care (Continued)

3. Effective date and durability. This Durable Power of Attorney is effective when two physicians decide and certify that I am incapacitated and unable to make and communicate a health care decision.

• If you want ONE physician, instead of TWO, to decide whether you are incapacitated, write your initials in the box to the right.

4. Agent's powers. I grant to my Agent full authority to:

A. Give consent to, prohibit, or withdraw any type of health care, medical care, treatment, or procedure, even if my death may result;

• If you wish to AUTHORIZE your Agent to direct a health care provider to withhold or withdraw artificially supplied nutrition and hydration (including tube feeding of food and water), write your initials in the box to the right.

• If you DO NOT WISH TO AUTHORIZE your Agent to direct a health care provider to withhold or withdraw artificially supplied nutrition and hydration (including tube feeding of food and water), write your initials in the box to the right.

B. Make all necessary arrangements for health care services on my behalf, and to hire and fire medical personnel responsible for my care;

C. Move me into or out of any health care facility (even if against medical advice) to obtain compliance with the decisions of my Agent; and

D. Take any other action necessary to do what I authorize here, including (but not limited to) granting any waiver or release from liability required by any health care provider, and taking any legal action at the expense of my estate to enforce this Durable Power of Attorney.

5. Agent's Financial Liability and Compensation. My Agent acting under this Durable Power of Attorney will incur no personal financial liability. My Agent shall not be entitled to compensation for services performed under this Durable Power of Attorney, but my Agent shall be entitled to reimbursement for all reasonable expenses incurred as a result of carrying out any provision hereof.

(continues)

Figure 7-3 *(continued)*

Reimbursement

Peer review organizations (PROs), consisting of physicians and nurses, are required by the federal government to monitor and evaluate the quality and appropriateness of care provided. Medical record documentation is the mechanism for the PRO review, which evaluates the intensity of services and the severity of illness on the basis of a comparison of sample medical records from different facilities against specific screening criteria.

The federal enactment of the diagnosis-related group (DRG) classification system changed the health care provider reimbursement process from a cost-per-case to a prospective payment system (PPS). With PPS, the medical record must provide documentation that supports the DRG and the appropriateness

---

Part II. Health Care Directive

• If you DO NOT WISH to make a health care directive, write your initials in the box to the right, and go to Part III.

☐ Initials

I make this HEALTH CARE DIRECTIVE ("Directive") to exercise my right to determine the course of my health care and to provide clear and convincing proof of my wishes and instructions about my treatment.

If I am persistently unconscious or there is no reasonable expectation of my recovery from a seriously incapacitating or terminal illness or condition, I direct that all of the life-prolonging procedures which I have initialed below be withheld or withdrawn.

I want the following life-prolonging procedures to be withheld or withdrawn:

• artificially supplied nutrition and hydration (including tube feeding of food and water) . . . . ☐ Initials

• surgery or other invasive procedures. . . . . ___ Initials

• heart-lung resuscitation (CPR) . . . . ___ Initials

• antibiotic. . . . . ___ Initials

• dialysis. . . . . ___ Initials

• mechanical ventilator (respirator). . . . . ___ Initials

• chemotherapy. . . . . ___ Initials

• radiation therapy. . . . . ___ Initials

• all other "life-prolonging" medical or surgical procedures that are merely intended to keep me alive without reasonable hope of improving my condition or curing my illness or injury. . . . . ___ Initials

However, if my physician believes that any life-prolonging procedure may lead to significant recovery, I direct my physician to try the treatment for a reasonable period of time. If it does not improve my condition, I direct the treatment be withdrawn even if it shortens my life. I also direct that I be given medical treatment to relieve pain or to provide comfort, even if such treatment might shorten my life, suppress my appetite or my breathing, or be habit forming.

IF I HAVE NOT DESIGNATED AN AGENT IN THE DURABLE POWER OF ATTORNEY, THIS DOCUMENT IS MEANT TO BE IN FULL FORCE AND EFFECT AS MY HEALTH CARE DIRECTIVE.

(continues)

Figure 7-3 *(continued)*

of care. Nursing documentation must also show evidence of client and family education and discharge planning.

From a hospital's perspective, when information in the medical record demonstrates compliance with Medicare and Medicaid standards, the reimbursement is maximized. If nurses fail to document the equipment or procedures used daily (e.g., feeding pump; daily weight, intake, and output; intravenous therapy; drug additives), reimbursement to the facility can be denied.

Another federal law, the Comprehensive Omnibus Budget Reconciliation Act (COBRA), allows employees to temporarily carry their employer-provided health insurance benefits for 90 days after termination, reduction in the work hours, or retirement. The law requires that for any COBRA client receiving care

---

Part III. General Provisions Included in the Directive and Durable Power of Attorney

YOU MUST SIGN THIS DOCUMENT IN THE PRESENCE OF TWO WITNESSES. IN WITNESS WHEREOF, I have executed this document this_____day of _____, year____.

_____
Signature

Print name _____
Address _____

The person who signed this document is of sound mind and voluntarily signed this document in our presence. Each of the undersigned witnesses is at least eighteen years of age.

Signature_____   Signature_____

Print name _____   Print name _____

Address _____   Address _____

ONLY REQUIRED FOR PART I — DURABLE POWER OF ATTORNEY

STATE OF MISSOURI   )

) as

_____OF _____   )

On this _____day of _____, year_____, before me personally appeared to me known to be the person described in and who executed the foregoing instrument and acknowledged that he/she executed the same as his/her free act and deed.

IN WITNESS WHEREOF, I have hereunto set my hand and affixed my official seal in the County of _____, State of Missouri, the day and year first above written.

_____
Notary Public

My Commision Expires:

Figure 7-3 *(continued)*

in an emergency room, the client's condition must be stabilized before the client can be transferred to another facility. If the client's condition is not stable, the institution cannot initiate a transfer.

Facilities in violation of COBRA laws are fined and stand to lose their eligibility for Medicare and Medicaid funding. Compliance with this law is evaluated through medical record review. The documentation concerning client transfers must include:

- Chronology of the event,
- Measures taken or treatment implemented,
- The client's response to treatment, and
- Results of measures taken to prevent the client's condition from deteriorating.

COMMUNITY/HOME HEALTH CARE

Documentation

Home health agencies also keep documents: physician's orders, history and physical form, home care team records, and nursing records (initial assessment form, plan of care, problem list for daily progress notes, client teaching activities, and discharge summary). Home health care providers are required to comply with state and federal regulations that affect health care, documentation, and reimbursement.

SUMMARY

- Documentation provides a system of written records that reflect client care provided on the basis of assessment data and the client's response to interventions.
- The medical record can be used by health care students as a teaching tool and is a main source of data for clinical research.
- Nurses are responsible for assessing and documenting that the client has an understanding of the treatment prior to the intervention.
- Accreditation and reimbursement agencies require accurate and thorough documentation of the nursing care rendered and the client's response to interventions.

Review Questions

1. Systematic documentation is critical because it:
   a. is done every hour.
   b. shows the care given by all health care providers.
   c. identifies the planning and implementation phases.
   d. presents in a logical fashion the care provided by nurses.

2. The two primary reasons for health care documentation are:
   a. education and research.
   b. research and reimbursement.
   c. accountability and responsibility.
   d. fulfillment of legal and practice standards.

3. The legal issues of documentation require the use of:
   a. black ink pens.
   b. legible, neat writing.
   c. short, descriptive phrases.
   d. hourly recording of client status.

4. The person responsible for obtaining a client's informed consent is the:
   a. physician.
   b. staff nurse.
   c. admissions clerk.
   d. nurse supervisor.

5. The person responsible for ensuring that the client understands the procedure or intervention and has signed the informed consent is the:
   a. nurse.
   b. physician.
   c. social worker.
   d. admission officer.

Critical Thinking Questions

1. Of what value is a client's medical record in a court of law? How can it be used?

2. Why should nurses know about reimbursement rules?

WEB FLASH!

- Check your state's board of nursing website for the nursing practice act.
- Search the Internet for information on advance directives.

References/Suggested Readings

Charting Tips. (1999). Documenting discharges and transfers in long-term care. *Nursing99, 29*(6), 17.

Eggland, E. T., & Heinemann, D. S. (1994). Nursing documentation: *Charting, recording, and reporting.* Philadelphia: Lippincott Williams & Wilkins.

Estes, M. E. Z. (2002). *Health assessment & physical examination* (2nd ed.). Albany, NY: Delmar.

Fiesta, J. (1991). If it wasn't charted, it was done! *Nursing Management, 22*(8), 17.

Glondys, B. (1999). *Documentation requirements for the acute care patient record.* Chicago, IL: American Health Information Management Association.

Grulke, C. C. (1995). Seven ways to help a student nurse. *AJN, 96*(60), 24L.

Iyer, P. W., & Camp, N. H. (1999). *Nursing documentation: A nursing process approach* (3rd ed.). St. Louis, MO: Mosby.

Joint Commission on Accreditation of Healthcare Organizations. (1998). *1998 Hospital accreditation standards.* Oakbrook Terrace, IL: Author.

LaDuke, S. (2000). Spotlight: What you *really* do with this powerful documentation tool. *Nursing2000, 30*(6), 68.

McConnell, E. (1999). Charting with care. *Nursing99, 29*(10), 68.

North American Nursing Diagnosis Association. (2001). *NANDA Nursing diagnoses: Definitions & classifications 2001–2002.* Philadelphia, PA: Author.

Olson-Chavarriaga, D. (2000). Informed consent: Do you know your role? *Nursing2000, 30*(5), 60–61.

Simmons, P. B., & Meadors, B. (1995). Eliminating friendly fire: Successful nursing documentation strategies. *Journal of Nursing Staff Development, 11*(2), 79–82.

Springhouse. (1999). *Mastering documentation* (2nd ed.). Springhouse, PA: Author.

Springhouse. (1998). *Charting made incredibly easy.* Springhouse, PA: Author.

Sullivan, G. (2000). Keep your charting on course. *RN, 63*(5), 75–79.

Tucker, J. L. (1995). Interdisciplinary record improves documentation. *Patient Education Management, 2*(3), 45–47.

White, L. (2001). *Foundations of nursing: Caring for the whole person.* Albany, NY: Delmar.

White, L. (2002). *Basic nursing: Foundations of skills & concepts.* Albany, NY: Delmar.

Resources

American Health Information Management Association
233 North Michigan Avenue, Suite 2150, Chicago, IL 60601-5800, 313-233-1100, www.ahima.org

CHAPTER 8

PRINCIPLES OF EFFECTIVE DOCUMENTATION

Upon completion of this chapter, you should be able to:
- *Discuss the elements of effective documentation.*
- *Describe how to document a medication error.*
- *Document client care effectively.*

INTRODUCTION

Documentation requirements differ depending on the health care facility (hospital, nursing home, home health agency), the setting within the facility (e.g., emergency room, perioperative unit, medical–surgical unit), and the specific client population (e.g., obstetric, pediatric, geriatric). Regardless of the client care administered, the documentation of that care must reflect the nursing process. General documentation guidelines are listed in Table 8-1.

FOLLOW THE NURSING PROCESS

Nursing notes must be logical, focused, and relevant to care and must represent each phase in the nursing process (Glondys, 1999; Habel 2000). Nursing documentation based on the nursing process facilitates effective care because client needs can be traced from assessment, through identification of the problems, to the care plan, implementation, and evaluation. A brief outline of the elements of the nursing process as they relate to documentation follows:

- *Assessment*: Assessment data related to an actual or potential health care need are summarized without duplication. With

Table 8-1   GENERAL DOCUMENTATION GUIDELINES

- Ensure that you have the correct client record or chart and that the client's name and identifying information are on every page of the record.

- Document as soon as the client encounter is concluded to ensure accurate recall of data (follow institutional guidelines on frequency of charting).

- Date and time each entry.

- Sign each entry with your full legal name and with your professional credentials, or per your institutional policy.

- Do not leave space between entries.

- If an error is made while documenting, use a single line to cross out the error, then date, time, and sign the correction (follow institutional policy); erasing, crossing out, or using correction fluid is not acceptable.

- Never change another person's entry, even if it is incorrect.

- The first entry of the shift should be made early (e.g., at 7:30 A.M. for the 7–3 shift, as opposed to 11:30 A.M. or 12 P.M.). Chart at least every 2 hours, or per institutional policy.

- Use quotation marks to indicate direct client responses (e.g., "I feel lousy").

- Document in chronologic order; if chronologic order is not used, state why.

- Write legibly.

- Use a permanent-ink pen (black is usually preferable because it photocopies well).

- Document in a complete but concise manner by using phrases and abbreviations as appropriate.

- Document all telephone calls that you make or receive that are related to a client's case.

Adapted from *Health Assessment & Physical Examination* (2nd ed.), by M. E. Z. Estes, 2002, Albany, NY: Delmar. Copyright 2002 by Delmar. Adapted with permission.

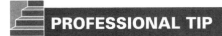

PROFESSIONAL TIP

Chart Following the Nursing Process

Charting in accordance with the nursing process ensures thorough documentation in compliance with nursing practice acts and with reimbursement and accreditation criteria.

reassessment, any new findings or any changes in the client's condition (e.g., increased pain) are highlighted.

- *Nursing diagnosis*: NANDA terminology to identify the client's problem or need.
- *Planning and outcome identification*: The expected client outcomes and goals, as discussed with the client and communicated to members of the multidisciplinary team, should be documented on the care plan or critical pathway rather than in the progress notes.
- *Implementation*: After an intervention has been performed, observations, treatments, teaching, and related clinical judgments should be documented on the flow sheet and progress notes. Client teaching should include learning needs, teaching plan content, methods of teaching, who was taught, and the client's response.
- *Evaluation*: The effectiveness of the interventions in terms of the expected outcomes is evaluated and documented: progress toward goals; client response to tests, treatments, and nursing interventions; client and family response to teaching and significant events; questions, statements, or problems voiced by the client or family.
- *Revisions of planned care*: The reasons for the revisions along with the supporting evidence and client agreement are documented.

ELEMENTS OF EFFECTIVE DOCUMENTATION

Several elements are important in producing effective documentation. To ensure effective documentation, nurses should:

- Document accurately, completely, and objectively including any errors that occurred

- Note date and time
- Use appropriate forms
- Identify the client
- Write in ink
- Use standard abbreviations
- Spell correctly
- Write legibly
- Correct errors properly
- Write on every line
- Chart omissions
- Sign each entry

Accurate, Complete, and Objective

Record just the facts—exactly what you see, hear, and do. For example, "Two 4 × 4s completely soaked with yellow-green drainage in 20 minutes" is more accurate than "large amount of drainage." Never record opinions or assumptions. Chart relevant information relating to client care and reflecting the nursing process (Figure 8-1). *Remember, if it is not charted, it was not done.* It is difficult to prove in court that an aspect of client care was provided if it was not documented.

Document information promptly; the information is more likely to be accurate and complete. Important details may be forgotten if charting is left until the end of the shift, and those details may later become a legal issue. Chart medications immediately *after* administration. This prevents errors such as another nurse administering pain medication when the first dose was not charted.

Avoid subjective statements such as "client is uncooperative." Record the client's exact words using quotation marks, for example, *Client stated, "I don't want to take a bath, and I don't want any breakfast."*

Date and Time

Be sure each entry is dated and has a specific time. Especially note the exact time of sudden changes in a client's condition, nursing actions, and other significant events. Do not chart in blocks of time, such as 7 A.M.–11 A.M. This is vague and sounds like the client has had no attention during that time frame.

NURSES' PROGRESS RECORD

DATE	HOUR	PROGRESS NOTES
2/3/02	0815	Client verbalizes severe abdominal pain (8 on a 0-10 pain scale). Lying on Right side. States "I don't want to take a bath, and I don't want any breakfast". Abdomen distended. No bowel sounds ascultated. Acute Pain R/T no flatus passed since surgery. ————————L. White, RN
2/3/02	0820	Administered Prostigmin Injection 0.5 mg (1 mL of 1:2000 solution) given IM in left gluteus maximus. Assisted to Left side (Sim's position). ————————L. White, RN
2/3/02	0900	Client states "I passed some gas, the pain is much less now, about a 4 (on 0-10 pain scale). ————————L. White, RN

Figure 8-1 Accurate, Complete, Objective Documentation

When military time is used, there is no confusion between A.M. and P.M. entries. For this reason many facilities use military time (Table 8-2).

Table 8-2 REGULAR AND MILITARY TIME

REGULAR TIME	MILITARY TIME	REGULAR TIME	MILITARY TIME
1 A.M.	0100	1 P.M.	1300
2 A.M.	0200	2 P.M.	1400
3 A.M.	0300	3 P.M.	1500
4 A.M.	0400	4 P.M.	1600
5 A.M.	0500	5 P.M.	1700
6 A.M.	0600	6 P.M.	1800
7 A.M.	0700	7 P.M.	1900
8 A.M.	0800	8 P.M.	2000
9 A.M.	0900	9 P.M.	2100
10 A.M.	1000	10 P.M.	2200
11 A.M.	1100	11 P.M.	2300
12 noon	1200	12 midnight	2400

If documentation cannot be done in a timely manner, explain the delay. For example, "chart in x-ray with client." When an entry must be added after notes are completed, follow the facility's policy for recording a late entry. Generally, the practice is to enter the date and time and note "Late Entry." This indicates that the entry is out of sequence. Then the date and time the entry should have been made is followed by the information to be recorded (Figure 8-2).

Use Appropriate Forms

Use the appropriate forms as required by the facility's policy manual. The forms used are not the same from facility to facility. Some facilities use flow sheets instead of progress notes.

Identify the Client

Each page of the client's record is to have the client's name on it. This aids in preventing confusion and helps ensure that information is charted on the correct record. Many facilities use the addressograph to stamp the client's name on each page.

Write in Ink

The client's record is a permanent document and information should be charted in ink or printed out from a computer. Only black ink should be used as it will photocopy well. Felt-tipped pens are not to be used, especially on forms with carbons since they do not hold up under pressure to make a clear copy. Also, they often bleed through the paper.

NURSES' PROGRESS RECORD

DATE	HOUR	PROGRESS NOTES
2/3/02	1100	Late Entry (2/3/02–0900) Client crying after talking to mother on the telephone.————————L. White, RN

Figure 8-2 Recording a Late Entry

Use Standard Abbreviations

Each health care facility has a list of approved abbreviations and symbols to be used in documenting information on their client records. This is to meet the Joint Commission on Accreditation of Healthcare Organization (JCAHO) standards and the regulations in many states. Such a list prevents confusion. The use of some abbreviations causes ambiguity that could be misleading and endanger a client's health (Figure 8-3).

Spell Correctly

Misspelled words on client records may be confusing and certainly convey a sense of unprofessionalism. They may generate questions about the quality of the care provided, increase the chance of liability, and produce a loss of credibility of the writer. When you are unsure of how to spell a word, *look it up.* Most units in a health care facility have a dictionary and other books to use as references.

Write Legibly

Legible handwriting is imperative for effective documentation. Sloppy writing hinders communication and possible errors in client care can occur. Trying to decipher illegible writing wastes time. Illegible handwriting creates a poor impression of the person who did the writing and damages that person's credibility. Print rather than use cursive writing; it is usually easier to read.

MEDICATION ADMINISTRATION RECORD

MEDICATION	DATE: 3/02/02		
	0701–1500	1501–2300	2301–0700
cyanocobalamin 20 Mg	*1400 LW*		

Shift	Signature	Initials
0701-1500	*L White RN*	*LW*
1501-2300		
2301-0700		

Is this milligram or microgram?

It is less confusing to use mcg for microgram.

Figure 8-3 Misleading Abbreviation

Correct Errors Properly

Promptly correct any error you make in documenting on a client's record. Know and follow your facility's policy for correcting errors. Generally, the following is accepted for charting errors. Draw a single line through the mistaken entry so that what was written can still be read. Carefully write above it "Mistaken Entry" followed by your initials and the date (Brooke, 2002; Pethtel, 2000; and Dumpel, James, & Phillips, 1999). The original entry must still be readable. *NEVER scratch out, erase, or use correction fluid (white-out)* on a mistaken entry. Using these methods makes it look like something is being hidden. Be sure the mistaken entry is still readable (Figure 8-4).

Write on Every Line

Fill each line completely. Leave no blank lines or partially blank lines. Draw a line through the empty part of the line (Figure 8-4). This prevents others from inserting information later that may change the meaning of the original documentation. On forms, when information requested does not apply to a particular client, write "NA" (not applicable) or draw a line through the space. This indicates that every item on the form has been addressed.

Chart Omissions

Charting is supposed to show implementation of the medical and nursing plans of care. Whenever a part of the plan is omit-

NURSES' PROGRESS RECORD

DATE	HOUR	PROGRESS NOTES
2/3/02	0600	Client verbalizes severe abdominal pain (8 on a 0–10 pain scale) when lying on ~~Left side~~ Right side.——L. White, RN

Figure 8-4 Mistaken Entry

ted, document the reason why. For example, a treatment was not provided or medication was not administered because the client was in x-ray (Figure 8-5).

Sign Each Entry

Each entry on the nurses notes (progress notes) is to be signed with your first name or initial, full last name, and professional licensure (i.e., LVN, LPN, RN). The signature should be at the end of the entry on the far right side. When there is not enough room on the last line of the documentation, draw a line from the last word to the end of the line and on the next line, leaving enough room to sign the entry at the far right.

For a long entry that will conclude on another page, record "(Continued on next page)" and sign your name. Begin the next page with "(Continued from previous page)," finish the entry, and sign your name (Figure 8-6).

NURSES' PROGRESS RECORD

DATE	HOUR	PROGRESS NOTES
2/3/02	0900	*Abdominal dressing not changed. Client in x-ray for a flat plate of the abdomen.* ——————— *L. White, RN*

Figure 8-5 Charting an Omitted Part of the Care Plan

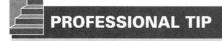

PROFESSIONAL TIP

Abbreviations

Avoid abbreviations that can be misunderstood. For example, what does the abbreviation *Pt* mean? Does it refer to the patient, prothrombin time, physical therapy, or part-time? Refer to your institution's approved abbreviations listing.

NURSES' PROGRESS RECORD

DATE	HOUR	PROGRESS NOTES
2/3/02	1300	to assess client's knowledge of diabetes (Continued on next
		page)————————————————L. White, RN

NURSES' PROGRESS RECORD

DATE	HOUR	PROGRESS NOTES
2/3/02	1300	(Continued from previous page) on the 3rd or 4th day
		post op————————————————L. White, RN

Figure 8-6 Entry Continues on Another Page

DOCUMENTING A MEDICATION ERROR

Facilities require nurses to report medication errors on incident reports (discussed below). The medication given in error should appear on the MAR and in the nurses' progress notes. It should be remembered that the purpose of the medical record is to report any care or treatment the client receives, including any errors made. However, no mention is made of an incident report being completed.

When a medication error occurs, the following documentation should be done:

- The medication should be charted on the MAR to prevent other caregivers from giving the client additional doses of the same drug, doses of similar drugs, or doses of drugs that may be contraindicated.
- The error should be documented in the nurses' notes with the following information: name and dosage of the medication; time it was given; client's response to the medication; name of the practitioner who was notified of the error; time of the notification; nursing interventions or medical treatment to counteract the error; and client's response to treatment.

Medication Incident Report

Some health care facilities are now using a specific medication incident (variance) report for situations related to medications (Figure 8-7). This provides the facility with information that can be used to possibly change policies or procedures that will work to prevent medication incidents.

Addressograph | *Addressograph*

CHRISTUS Health
QUALITY COMMITTEE
Medication Safety And Quality Report
Adverse Drug Event(Errors/Reactions)
Medical Record #:
☐ Male ☐ Female
Name:

Address:

Medication Error: any preventable event that may cause or lead to inappropriate medication use or patient harm, including prescribing, order communication, product labeling, packaging, compounding, dispensing, distribution, administration and use. (adapted from USP); any variance from the established process.

Instructions: Person discovering event completes Sections 1 through 13 according to facility policy and procedure. Forward to manager for additional review and investigation. Manager or analyst completes sections 14 through 19.

Event Number:__________ **(# assigned by Risk Management)** **1. Diagnosis:**

2. FACILITY NAME ____________________ **3. Date of Occurrence** : ___/___/___ Time ___:___ AM PM

4. Event Type: Variance Occurred to: ☐ Patient(01) ☐ Other(OT) **Check if event occurred on:** ☐ Holiday ☐ Weekends

5. Type/Event Indicator:

☐ Adverse Drug Reaction	(70.10)	☐ Monitoring Error	(70.60)	☐ Wrong Rate	(77.10)
☐ Deteriorated Drug Errors (dispensing expired drug)	(70.20)	☐ Clinical (lab, vital signs)	(70.61)	☐ Too Fast	(71.11)
☐ Dose Omission	(70.30)	☐ Documented Allergy	(70.62)	☐ Too Slow	(71.12)
☐ Improper Dose	(70.40)	☐ Drug-Disease Interaction	(70.63)	☐ Wrong Route of Administration:	(71.20)
☐ Extra Dose	(70.41)	☐ Drug-Drug Interaction	(70.64)	☐ Wrong Strength/Concentration	(71.30)
☐ Frequency	(70.42)	☐ Drug-Food/ Interaction	(70.65)	☐ Wrong Technique	(71.40)
☐ Resulting in Overdosage	(70.43)	☐ Narcotic Discrepancy	(71.60)	☐ Wrong Time	(71.50)
☐ Resulting in Under Dosage	(70.44)	☐ Wrong Dosage Form	(70.70)	☐ Other	(79.99)
☐ IV Infiltration/Extravasation	(70.50)	☐ Wrong Drug	(70.80)		
		☐ Wrong Duration	(70.90)		
		☐ Wrong Patient	(70.00)		

6. Setting of initial event:(Dept. or unit) **7. Setting where event discovered: (Dept or unit)**

8. Medication as Ordered: (Name, Dose, Route, Frequency) **9. Medication as Dispensed or Administered:**

10. DESCRIPTION OF EVENT:

11. Patient Outcome: (Errors or reactions with ** to left of description require physician notification and notification of Risk Management according to facility policy and procedure)

- ☐ No Error, but circumstances, policies or procedures that could lead to error (31.0)
- ☐ Error occurred but medication did not reach patient.(i.e. dispensing error, caught in pharmacy or on delivery to unit) (32.1)
- ☐ Error or reaction that reaches patient (32.2)
  - ☐ Medication reaches the patient but not administered (32.4)
  - ☐ ** Medication reaches the patient and is administered, no additional treatment, monitoring or intervention (32.3)
- ☐ ** Increased patient monitoring only(more frequent vital signs, laboratory tests ordered) (32.5)
- ☐ ** Treatment or intervention required(meds ordered, procedures required) (33.1)
- ☐ **Initial or prolonged hospitalization (33.2)
- ☐ ** Permanent patient harm (33.3)
- ☐ ** Near-death event (e.g., anaphylaxis, cardiac arrest) (33.4)
- ☐ **Death (34.0)

12. Reported By: __________ Date: __/__/__ Time: __:__ AM PM Risk Mgmt notified? ☐ Yes ☐ No

13. Physician Notified ☐ Yes ☐ No By: __________ Date: __/__/__ Time: __:__ AM PM

THIS IS A COMMITTEE DOCUMENT & IS PRIVILEGED AND CONFIDENTIAL.

(continues)

Figure 8-7 Medication Incident Report (Courtesy of CHRISTUS Spohn Hospital Shoreline, Corpus Christi, TX)

Sections 14 through 19 to be completed by Manager

14. Persons Involved (include name and phone, if appropriate, for purpose of followup or participation in possible root cause analysis)

Ordered Med: _____   ☐ Intern (A1)   ☐ Resident(A2)   ☐ Other Physician(A3)
☐ Nurse Practitioner/Advanced Practice (C1)

Prepared/Administered Med: _____   ☐ Registered Nurse(C2)   ☐ Licensed Practical Nurse(C3)
☐ Pharmacy Technician (E)   ☐ Pharmacist (B)
☐ Other(H) _____

Dispensed Med: _____   ☐ Pharmacist (B)   ☐ Other(H) _____

15. **System Breakdown Points: Were any of the following items identified during error investigation? Check all that apply**

☐ Administration not documented	(C1)	☐ Location(adjacent medications)	(C27)
☐ Allergy information not in chart	(C2)	☐ Look alike/Sound alike product name/packaging	(C28)
☐ Allergy information not on MAR/Kardex	(C3)	☐ Look alike/Sound alike patient name	(C29)
☐ Armband/name not checked	(C4)	☐ MAR/Kardex incorrect, misleading or unclear	(C30)
☐ Abbreviations	(C5)	☐ Medication not available at scheduled admin time	(C31)
☐ Automated dispensing device	(C6)	☐ Medication stored in wrong drawer/location	(C32)
☐ Calculation error in pharmacy	(C7)	☐ Multiple orders for same medication	(C33)
☐ Calculation error on nursing unit	(C8)	☐ Order entry error (user error)	(C18)
☐ Change of shift	(C9)	☐ Order not sent to/received by pharmacy	(C34)
☐ Computer system down	(C10)	☐ Order overlooked/missed by pharmacy	(C35)
☐ Computer system functionality	(C50)	☐ Order overlooked/missed by nursing	(C36)
☐ Decimal error(NOT Leading/Trailing Zeros)	(C11)	☐ Order misinterpreted by pharmacy	(C37)
☐ Delayed dose	(C12)	☐ Order misinterpreted by nursing	(C49)
☐ Documentation	(C17)	☐ Order stamped/labeled for wrong patient	(C19)
☐ Error in stocking/restocking/cart fill/floor stock etc	(C13)	☐ Order unclear or ambiguous	(C38)
☐ Handwriting	(C14)	☐ Patient off unit	(C39)
☐ Illegible fax or NCR order copy	(C15)	☐ Patient with stated allergy to medication given	(C40)
☐ Incomplete order	(C16)	☐ Policy/procedure not followed	(C41)
☐ Insufficient staff	(C20)	☐ Prepared in patient care area	(C42)
☐ Inexperienced staff	(C21)	☐ Pump programmed incorrectly	(C43)
☐ Fatigue or extended shift	(C22)	☐ Pump/Equipment failure	(C44)
☐ Lack of training	(C23)	☐ Transfer patient /orders	(C45)
☐ Leading/Trailing zeros	(C24)	☐ Transcription error	(C46)
☐ Labeling of drug incorrect or misleading	(C25)	☐ Verbal order	(C47)
☐ Lack of knowledge	(C26)	☐ Other (Explain in section 16)	(C48)

16. **Notes regarding investigation, action, recommendations for system improvement:**

_____
_____
_____
_____

17. **Nature of Injury:** (Check all that apply)			
☐ Abscess (04)	☐ Blood Disorder (62)	☐ Hearing Disorder (39)	☐ Respiratory Disorder/	☐ Tissue Damage (61)
☐ Amputation (06)	☐ Circulatory Impairment (11)	☐ Heart Attack (41)	Asphyxia/Choking (43)	☐ Visual Impairment (40)
☐ Anoxia (44)	☐ Dermatitis/Skin Disorder(29)	☐ Hematoma (51)	☐ Rupture (59)	☐ Other (99)
☐ Blister (50)	☐ Deterioration in Condition(14)	☐ Infection (31)	☐ Seizure (22)	
	☐ Fever (24)	☐ Inflammation (27)	☐ Shock (Non-Electrical) (37)	
	☐ Headache (52)	☐ Phlebitis (19)	☐ Stroke (45)	☐ No Injury Noted (48)

18. **Does this injury involve one of these outcomes...** (Check only one)			
☐ Amputation (01)	☐ Burn (04)	☐ Loss of Hearing (13)	☐ Residual Paralysis (18)
☐ Birth Injury (02)	☐ Events Resulting in Disability (06)	☐ Loss of Eyesight (12)	☐ Septicemia After Admission (19)
☐ Brain Damage (03)	☐ Kidney Failure (11)	☐ Loss of Sensation (14)	☐ Unexpected Death (20)

19. Manager Review: _____   Date: _____

20. Director: Administrator Review: _____   Date: _____

THIS IS A COMMITTEE DOCUMENT & IS PRIVILEGED AND CONFIDENTIAL.

Figure 8-7 *(continued)*

SUMMARY

- Effective documentation requires clear, concise, accurate recording of all client care and other significant events in an organized and chronologic fashion representative of each phase of the nursing process.
- Use only agency approved abbreviations.
- Add a late entry or correct a mistaken entry following the agency-approved method.

- Sign *each* entry appropriately.
- Client safety requires appropriate reporting and recording of medication errors and other occurrences, in compliance with the facility's policy.

Review Questions

1. Documentation of the nursing care the client receives must:
   a. never have an error.
   b. be neatly spaced out.
   c. reflect the nursing process.
   d. be signed only at the end of each shift.

2. A medication error is documented on the:
   a. graphic sheet.
   b. nursing plan of care.
   c. health care team record.
   d. medication administration record.

3. When a documentation error has been made, it should:
   a. be erased.
   b. be scratched out.
   c. have one line drawn through it.
   d. be whited out so as to keep the record neat.

4. When documenting client care, abbreviations and symbols:
   a. may not be used.
   b. approved by the facility may be used.
   c. should be used very sparingly, one per page.
   d. approved by the medical society and the nursing organization may be used.

Critical Thinking Questions

1. Why are nursing notes to include each component of the nursing process?

2. Why is a medication error to be documented on the MAR and in the nurses notes?

WEB FLASH!

- Search the web for documenting client care. What helpful hints are found?
- What information is found on the Internet about documenting a medication error?

References/Suggested Readings

Brooke, P. (2002). Legal questions: Documentation errors. *Nursing2002, 32*(1), 67.

DeWitt, A. (2000). *Documentation: Legal principles of good charting.* Penumbra Seminars LLC [On-line]. Available: www.respiratorycare-online.com/doc_handoutPDF

Dumpel, H., James, M., & Phillips, T. (1999). Charting by exception. *California Nurse*, June/July 1999, p. 9 [On-line]. Available: www.califnurses.org/cna/cal/junju99/9cnjj99.html

Eggland, E. T., & Heinemann, D. S. (1994). *Nursing documentation: Charting, recording, and reporting.* Philadelphia: Lippincott Williams & Wilkins.

Estes, M. E. Z. (2002). *Health assessment & physical examination* (2nd ed.). Albany, NY: Delmar.

Fiesta, J. (1991). If it wasn't charted, it was done! *Nursing Management, 22*(8), 17.

Glondys, B. (1999). *Documentation requirements for the acute care patient record.* Chicago, IL: American Health Information Management Association.

Habel, M. (2000a). *Documenting patient care, Part 1* [On-line]. Available: www.nurseweek.com/cc/ce10a.html

Habel, M. (2000b). *Documenting patient care, Part 2* [On-line] Available: www.nurseweek.com/cc/ce20a.html

Iyer, P. W., & Camp, N. H. (1999). *Nursing documentation: A nursing process approach* (3rd ed.). St. Louis, MO: Mosby.

Joint Commission on Accreditation of Healthcare Organizations. (1998). *1998 Hospital accreditation standards.* Oakbrook Terrace, IL: Author.

McCloskey, J. C., & Bulechek, G. M. (1994). Standardizing the language for nursing treatments: An overview of the issues. *Nursing Outlook, 42*(2), 56–63.

McConnell, E. (1999). Charting with care. *Nursing99, 29*(10), 68.

North American Nursing Diagnosis Association. (2001). *NANDA Nursing diagnoses: Definitions & classifications 2001–2002.* St. Louis, MO: Author.

Pethtel, P. (2000). *Nursing documentation* [On-line]. Available: http://garnet.indstate.edu/ppethtel/chartingforweb/

Simmons, P. B., & Meadors, B. (1995). Eliminating friendly fire: Successful nursing documentation strategies. *Journal of Nursing Staff Development, 11*(2), 79–82.

Springhouse. (1998). *Charting made incredibly easy.* Springhouse, PA: Springhouse.

Springhouse. (1999). *Mastering documentation* (2nd ed.). Springhouse, PA: Author.

Sullivan, G. (2000). Keep your charting on course. *RN, 63*(5), 75–79.

Thompson, C. (1995). Writing better narrative notes. *Nursing95, 25*(5), 87.

White, L. (2001). *Foundations of nursing: Caring for the whole person.* Albany, NY: Delmar.

White, L. (2002). *Basic nursing: Foundations of skills & concepts.* Albany, NY: Delmar.

CHAPTER

METHODS OF
DOCUMENTATION

LEARNING OBJECTIVES

Upon completion of this chapter, you should be able to:
- *Define key terms.*
- *Compare the various methods of documentation.*
- *Appropriately document client care following the facility's method of documentation.*

KEY TERMS

charting by exception
critical pathway
focus charting
narrative charting
PIE charting

point-of-care charting
problem-oriented medical
   record
source-oriented charting
variance

INTRODUCTION

Throughout the development of modern nursing, multiple documentation systems have emerged in response to changes in health care delivery. Systems of recording and reporting data pertinent to the care of clients have evolved primarily in response to the demand that health care practitioners be held to societal norms, professional standards of practice, legal and regulatory standards, and institutional policies and standards.

As with all facets of health care, advanced technology has affected the expectations for documentation. Activities in the areas of quality improvement and cost containment have also increased the demands on health care practitioners to create efficient documentation systems. Efficiency is measured in terms of time, thoroughness, and the quality of the observations being recorded. The documentation systems used today reflect the specific needs and preferences of the numerous health care agencies. Select systems and their ramifications are discussed in this chapter.

Documentation must reflect the complexity of care and must embody accuracy, completeness, and evidence of professional practice. The clinical standards (structure, outcome, process, and evaluation) are used to develop a system that complies with legal, accreditation, and professional practice requirements of documentation.

Among the many methods used for documentation are the following:

• Narrative charting
• Source-oriented charting
• Problem-oriented charting
• PIE charting
• Focus charting
• Charting by exception
• Computerized documentation
• Critical pathways

NARRATIVE CHARTING

Narrative charting, the traditional method of nursing documentation, is a chronologic account written in paragraphs describing the client's status, interventions, and treatments, and the client's response to treatments. Before the advent of flow sheets, this was the only method for documenting care.

Narrative documentation is the most flexible of all methods and is usable in any clinical setting. The relationship between nursing interventions and client's responses is clearly shown. The chronologic order allows team members to review client progress each day (Figure 9-1).

With this type of documentation, however, subjectivity is a common problem. Client problems may be difficult to track because the same information may not be consistently documented. The client's progress may be difficult to identify. Often narrative charting fails to reflect the nursing process.

NURSES' PROGRESS RECORD

DATE	HOUR	PROGRESS NOTES
2/3/02	1630	Client 6 hours post op; awakens easily, oriented x 3.
		Abdominal dressing dry and intact. Denies pain but stated he
		felt nauseated and immediately vomited 50 mL of clear fluid.
		Attempted to ambulate to bathroom with assistance, but felt
		dizzy. Assisted to lie down in bed. Voided 250 mL clear, yel-
		low urine in urinal. Client encouraged to turn in bed, cough,
		and deep breathe.————————————L. White, RN
2/3/02	1650	Continues to feel nauseated. Tigan 250 mg given by
		mouth.————————————L. White, RN
2/3/02	1730	States he is no longer nauseated. Remains pain free.
		Properly demonstrated coughing and deep breathing.——
		————————————L. White, RN

Figure 9-1 Narrative Charting

SOURCE-ORIENTED CHARTING

Source-oriented charting is described as a narrative recording on separate sheets by each member (source) of the health care team. Because each discipline uses a separate sheet, care is often fragmented, and communication between disciplines is time-consuming. Source-oriented charting has similar advantages and disadvantages to narrative charting, because both methods take an unstructured approach to documenting in the progress notes.

PROBLEM-ORIENTED CHARTING

Problem-oriented medical record (POMR) focuses on the client's problem and employs a structured, logical format.

There are four critical components of POMR/POR:

- Database (assessment data)
- Problem list (client's problems numbered according to when identified)
- Initial plan (outline of goals, expected outcomes, learning needs and further data, if needed)
- Progress notes (charting based on the SOAP, SOAPIE, or SOAPIER format)

A prominent feature is the format in which progress notes are to be written (i.e., SOAP, SOAPIE, SOAPIER).

- S: subjective data (what the client or family member states)
- O: objective data (what is observed/inspected)
- A: assessment (conclusion reached on the basis of data formulated as client problem or nursing diagnosis)
- P: plan (expected outcome and actions to be taken)

SOAPIE and SOAPIER refer to formats that add the following:

- I: intervention (measures taken to achieve expected outcomes)
- E: evaluation (analyze effectiveness of interventions)
- R: revision (changes in original plan)

An entry need not be made for each component of SOAP(IER) at every documentation (Figure 9-2). However, each problem must have a complete note every 24 hours if unresolved or whenever the client's condition changes. The structured format makes communication between health care team members easier. Continuity of care is shown when the plan of care and interventions performed are documented together. Figure 9-2 shows an example of SOAPIE charting. Some physicians use this format when writing progress notes.

PIE CHARTING

After the SOAP format gained popularity, the Problem, Intervention, Evaluation **(PIE) charting** system evolved to streamline documentation. The key components of this system are assessment flow sheets, nurses' progress notes, and an integrated plan of care. Figure 9-3 shows an example of PIE charting. This system eliminates the traditional care plan by incorporating an ongoing plan of care (problem, intervention, evaluation) into the daily documentation.

FOCUS CHARTING

Focus charting is a documentation method that uses a column format to chart data, action, and response (DAR) (Smith,

NURSES' PROGRESS RECORD

DATE	HOUR	PROGRESS NOTES
2/3/02	0730	#1 Pain
		S: Client states "The pain in my hip is so bad."
		O: Client states pain is 9 (0–10 scale); skin warm, moist,
		pale. Lying stiffly in bed with fists clenched.
		A: Acute Pain, needs medication for relief
		P: Check orders for analgesia; check vital signs; if within
		normal limits give analgesia as ordered; then recheck in 30
		minutes for response.———————————L. White, RN
2/3/02	0740	#1 Pain
		O: BP 142/86, P 104, R 28
		I: meperidine 75 mg IM in right gluteus maximus.———
		————————————————L. White, RN
2/3/02	0810	#1 Pain
		S: Client states "The pain is better."
		O: Client states pain now 4 (0–10 scale); skin warm, dry,
		normal color. Lying relaxed in bed.
		A: Pain relieved
		P: Continue to monitor for pain
		E: Analgesic effective————————L. White, RN
2/3/02	0810	#2 Anxiety
		S: Client states "I'm still worried about the surgery on my
		hip."
		O: Client clutching sheet
		A: Anxiety R/T surgery the next day
		P: Encourage verbalization of concerns and feelings. Involve
		family in discussion of concerns, if client agreeable.———
		————————————————L. White, RN

Figure 9-2 SOAPIE Charting

2000). Usually the focus is a nursing diagnosis, but it may refer to:

- a sign or symptom (i.e., abnormal vaginal bleeding)
- an acute change in the client's condition (i.e., sudden increase in blood pressure)
- a special need (i.e., a discharge referral)

NURSES' PROGRESS RECORD

DATE	HOUR	PROGRESS NOTES
2/3/02	0830	P #1: Disturbed Body Image R/T bilateral mastectomy—
		I #1: Encourage verbalization of feelings and concerns and
		remain alert for client's comments about body changes;
		encourage looking at surgical site when ready—
		E #1: Glanced at chest during dressing change. Continue
		encouraging client's involvement in dressing changes.—
		——————————————————L. White, RN
2/3/02	0830	P #2: Ineffective Breathing Pattern R/T musculoskele-
		tal impairment following mastectomy—
		I #2: Encourage use of incentive spirometer every 2 hours
		increasing level each day; assess breath sounds, rate, and
		quality of respirations every 4 hours; monitor O₂ saturation
		with pulse oximeter—
		E #2: Using incentive spirometer every 2 hours when
		awake. Breath sounds normal, respirations 20 shallow, O₂
		saturation 93%.——————————L. White, RN

Figure 9-3 PIE Charting

Data includes subjective and objective information describing the focus. Action includes immediate and future nursing actions. Response is the client's response to the nursing actions (Figure 9-4). The column format of focus charting is used within the progress notes to distinguish the entry from other recordings in the narrative notes, as shown in Figure 9-4.

CHARTING BY EXCEPTION

Charting by exception (CBE) is a documentation method using standardized protocols stating what the expected course of the illness is and only significant findings (exceptions) are documented in a narrative form. It assumes that client care needs are routine and predictable and that the client's responses and outcomes are also routine and predictable.

The rule of thumb related to charting "if it is not charted, it was not done" is replaced in CBE by the presumption that unless documented otherwise, all standardized protocols have been met and no further documentation is needed. Time spent by nurses documenting client care may be reduced, but accord-

NURSES' PROGRESS RECORD

DATE	HOUR	FOCUS	PROGRESS NOTES
2/3/02	1300	Deficient	D: Client states that she does not
		Knowledge R/T	understand why she has to take three
		medications	medications. "I don't like to take pills."
			A: Reason for each medication explained,
			dosages, and side effects.
			R: Client verbalizes better understanding
			of her medications. ——L. White, RN
2/3/02	1600	Abnormal	D: Client states that her period just
		vaginal bleeding	started and she is passing clots.
			A: One maxi pad saturated in 30 minutes.
			BP 110/68, P 100, R 20. No clots seen.
			Status reported to Dr. Medoffer and
			orders received. IV started with 20 G
			catheter, 1000 mL normal saline hung at
			100 mL/h. Continue monitoring bleeding
			and vital signs. Dr. Medoffer will see
			client in 1 hour.
			R: Client understands reason for IV.——
			——L. White, RN

Figure 9-4 Focus Charting

ing to Dumpel, James, & Phillips (1999), charting by exception is not in the best interest of the client, and according to DeWitt (2000), charting by exception is a ticket to the courtroom.

COMPUTERIZED CHARTING

Health care facilities have been using computers for many years to order diagnostic tests and medications and to receive results of diagnostic tests. Nurses actually documenting client assessments, care plans, nursing interventions, and evaluations on a computerized client record has been much slower in being adopted. It takes a huge commitment for a facility, both financial and time, to plan for and make the change to computerized client records.

Issues to be addressed when considering computerized client records include data standards, vocabularies, security, legal issues, and costs.

- Data Standards—include length of fields, how dates and times are shown and ASCII or binary data.
- Vocabularies—the most commonly used are the combination of North American Nursing Diagnosis Association (NANDA) nursing diagnoses, Nursing Interventions Classification (NIC) nursing interventions, and Nursing Outcomes Classification (NOC) nursing outcomes.
- Security—includes privacy, confidentiality, who has access to which data, how errors are to be corrected, and protection against data loss.
- Legal Issues—electronic signatures
- Costs—include planning, hardware, software, and training for all users.

Nursing information systems (NIS) are various software programs that allow nursing documentation in an electronic record. These systems generally follow the components of the nursing process. The NIS works in conjunction with the hospital information system (HIS). Each NIS can be customized to fit a facility's documentation forms.

Decision-support systems are available to alert nurses, physicians, and pharmacists of client drug incompatibility, appropriate antibiotics based on culture and antibiotic susceptibility results, and adverse drug reactions. Another decision-support system uses assessment data to suggest possible nursing diagnoses, goals and outcome criteria, and interventions from which the nurse selects those appropriate for a specific client.

Bedside computer terminals allow the nurse to immediately document client assessments, medications given, and interventions performed; also the nurse can check care plans and revise if necessary, check test results, and many other functions. Timeliness, completeness, and the quality of nursing documentation are improved.

Voice-activated systems are available in some facilities. The nurse speaks into a special telephone handset and the words appear on the computer screen. These are generally at a central place rather than at the bedside.

Besides reducing documentation time and increasing accuracy, computerized charting increases legibility; stores and retrieves information quickly and easily; helps link diverse sources of client information; and uses standardized terminology, thus improving communication among health care departments. Planners for health care, researchers, lawyers, and third-party payers can quickly and easily retrieve information for their respective jobs.

Problems with computerized charting may occur if used incorrectly and client information may be mixed up. When security measures are neglected, client confidentiality may be compromised. Users (nurses, physicians, etc.) should never share computer ID numbers or passwords with anyone. Many systems keep a record of what each user has done in the system.

To prevent these problems, users must also remember to log off to prevent the unauthorized access of others. Users should also follow facility protocol for correcting errors, and keep monitors and print versions of client information where others cannot see the information (Habel, 2000b).

Information is temporarily unavailable when the computer system is "down" either for routine servicing or an unexpected failure. Processing time may be slow during peak usage times when too few terminals are available.

POINT-OF-CARE CHARTING

Point-of-care charting is a computerized documentation system that allows health care practitioners to have immediate access to client information. The system allows for the input and retrieval of client data at the bedside through a handheld portable computer. This is especially useful for nurses working in home health care.

The advantages of point-of-care charting relate to the efficiency of the computer system. Because this documentation method allows health care practitioners to record client data at the point of care:

• Operating costs are controlled
• Existing information systems are complemented
• Redundant data entry is eliminated
• The practitioner has more one-on-one time for client care, and
• Crucial client information is available to the health care practitioner in a timely fashion.

Point-of-care computerized documentation focuses on the continuum of care. Each health care practitioner is provided with all pertinent client data to ensure continuity of care without duplication. Point-of-care charting fosters compliance with accreditation and regulatory standards.

Disadvantages include all the problems inherent in computerized storage of records, such as maintaining confidentiality, controlling who has access to which data, and correcting errors.

CRITICAL PATHWAY

A **critical pathway** (care map) is a comprehensive preprinted interdisciplinary standard plan of care reflecting the ideal course of treatment for the average client with a given diagnosis or procedure, especially those with relatively predictable outcomes. They are generally not written for extremely complex client situations with less predictable outcomes.

The overall goal for critical pathways is to improve the quality and efficiency of client care. The sequence and timing of interdisciplinary activities is established including assessments, consultations, diagnostic tests, nutrition, medications, activities, treatments, therapeutics, education, and discharge planning (Figure 9-5). While nursing diagnoses as such are not generally included in a critical pathway, a nurse may identify nursing diagnoses and interventions for a specific client. For example, a client who had an appendectomy two days ago now has severe abdominal pain.

Health care facilities develop their own critical pathways. An interdisciplinary team including nurses, physicians, dietary, rehabilitative services, social services, and others when needed, develop the critical pathway through consensus about the management of the identified case situation. This is a time consuming task; but once written, a critical pathway can be revised based on a review of the variances.

Variances are goals not met or interventions not performed according to the established time frame. The nurse documents on a variance form why a goal is not met or an intervention is not performed (Klenner, 2000).

Critical pathways allow for the efficient use of time and increase the quality of care by having the expected outcomes identified on the plan. When clients have more than two diagnoses or variations, however, documentation becomes complicated because of limited space. This situation requires additional documentation forms to complement the pathway, such as intervention flow sheets and nurses' notes.

Sample Critical Pathway

PNEUMONIA

Expected stay 5 days

	Date:_____ Day 1	Date:_____ Day 2	Date:_____ Day 3
Assessments	Vital signs q 4 hr	Vital signs q 4 hr	Intake and Output
	Respiratory status: breath sounds and effort q 4 hr	Respiratory status: breath sounds and effort q 4 hr	When awake: Vital signs q 4 hr Respiratory status q 4 hr
	Pulse oximetry q 4 hr	Pulse oximetry q 4 hr	Pulse oximetry q 4 hr
	Intake and Output	Intake and Output	
Diagnostic Tests	CBC with differential	ABGs	Check blood culture report
	ABGs		Check sputum C&S report
	Blood culture x 2		Chest x-ray
	Sputum for gram stain and C&S		
	Chest x-ray		
Nutrition	As tolerated with small, nutritionally balanced, frequent meals. Encourage fluid intake to 2000 mL unless contraindicated.	As tolerated with small, nutritionally balanced, frequent meals. Encourage fluid intake to 2000–3000 mL unless contraindicated.	As tolerated with small, nutritionally balanced, frequent meals. Encourage fluid intake to 2000–3000 mL unless con-traindicated.

(continues)

Figure 9-5 Sample Critical Pathway

	Day 1	Day 2	Day 3
Medications	Oxygen as ordered to maintain O_2 saturation greater than 95%. IV fluids as ordered. IV antibiotics as ordered. Bronchodilators as ordered. Acetominophen 650 mg q 4 hr pain or fever over 101. Laxative of choice PRN.	Oxygen as ordered to maintain O_2 saturation greater than 95%. IV fluids as ordered. IV antibiotics as ordered. Bronchodilators as ordered. Acetominophen 650 mg q 4 hr pain or fever over 101. Laxative of choice PRN.	Oxygen as ordered to maintain O_2 saturation greater than 95%. D/C IV fluids. D/C IV antibiotics. Bronchodilators as ordered. Acetominophen 650 mg q 4 hr pain or fever over 101. Laxative of choice PRN.
Activity	Position in semi-Fowler's or high Fowler's position. Assess safety needs and provide appropriate precautions. Bathroom with assistance. Assist with ADLs. Provide rest periods.	Position in semi-Fowler's or high Fowler's position. Maintain safety precautions. Bathroom with assistance. Ambulate in room with assistance. Assist with ADLs. Provide rest periods.	Position in semi-Fowler's or high Fowler's position. Maintain safety precautions. Bathroom with assistance. Ambulate 4 times with assistance. Assist with ADLs. Provide rest periods.

(continues)

Figure 9-5 *(continued)*

	Day 1	Day 2	Day 3
Treatments	Incentive spriometer q 2 hr Nebulizer therapy q 4 hr Chest physical therapy Postural drainage 3 x/day Turn, cough, deep breathe q 1–2 hr	Incentive spirometer q 2 hr Nebulizer therapy q 4 hr Chest physical therapy Postural drainage 3 x/day Turn, cough, deep breathe q 1–2 hr	Incentive spirometer q 2 hr Nebulizer therapy q 4 hr Chest physical therapy Postural drainage 3 x/day Turn, cough, deep breathe q 1–2 hr
Education	Orient to room and facility routine. Review plan of care. Teach: cover mouth and nose when coughing or sneezing, dispose of tissues in trash bag. Evaluate understanding of teaching. Include family/ significant other.	Review plan of care. Evaluate understanding of teaching: increased fluids; rest/activity; turn, cough, deep breathe; incentive spirometer. Begin smoking cessation teaching (if client uses nicotine). Evaluate understanding of teaching. Include family/ significant other.	Reinforce earlier teaching. Begin discharge teaching: diet, rest, activity. Evaluate understanding of teaching. Include family/ significant other.

(continues)

Figure 9-5 *(continued)*

	Day 1	Day 2	Day 3
Discharge Planning	Establish discharge goals with client and family.	Review progress toward goals. Identify possible referrals.	Review progress toward goals.

	Date:_____	Date:_____
	Day 4	Day 5
Assessments	Routine vital signs Respiratory status each shift. Pulse oximetry each shift. Intake and output.	Routine vital signs Respiratory status each shift. Pulse oximetry each shift. Intake and output.
Diagnostic Tests		ABGs Chest x-ray
Nutrition	As tolerated with small, nutritionally balanced, frequent meals. Encourage fluid intake to 3000 mL unless contraindicated.	As tolerated with small, nutritionally balanced, frequent meals. Encourage fluid intake to 3000 mL unless contraindicated.
Medications	D/C oxygen if O_2 saturation 98% on room air. D/C IV antibiotics and IV fluids. Antibiotics orally as ordered. Bronchodilators as ordered. Acetominophen 650 mg q 4 hr PRN pain or fever over 101.	Antibiotics as ordered. Bronchodilators as ordered. Acetominophen 650 mg q 4 hr PRN pain or fever over 101.

(continues)

Figure 9-5 *(continued)*

	Day 4	Day 5
Activity	Maintain safety precautions. Ambulate independently at least 4 times.	Ambulatory
Treatments	Incentive spirometer q 2 hr. Nebulizer therapy q 4 hr. Chest physical therapy. Postural drainage 3 x/day. Turn, cough, deep breathe q 1–2 hr.	Incentive spirometer q 2 hr. Nebulizer therapy q 4 hr. Chest physical therapy. Turn, cough, deep breathe q 1–2 hr.
Education	Reinforce earlier teaching. Review written discharge instructions with client/family. Evaluate understanding of teaching.	Reinforce earlier teaching. Provide written discharge instructions. Finish discharge teaching including: diet; signs and symptoms to report; activity; medications: name, purpose, dose, frequency, route, side effects, dietary interactions; and follow-up physician visit. Evaluate understanding of teaching.
Discharge	Review progress toward goals. Finalize discharge plans.	Make referrals as identified. Complete discharge teaching.

Figure 9-5 *(continued)*

SUMMARY

- Narrative charting requires an organized, chronologic presentation of the client's problems and responses to interventions.
- Problem-oriented charting provides structure when documenting the client's problems and responses in the nurses' progress notes.
- Computerized documentation saves time, increases legibility and accuracy, provides standardized nursing terminology, enhances the nursing process and decision-making skills, and supports continuity of care.
- Critical pathways are comprehensive, standard plans of care for specific cases with predictable outcomes. Only variances are documented.

Review Questions

1. An advantage of the narrative charting format is it:
  a. uses flow charts.
  b. is the most flexible of all methods.
  c. clearly tracks trends and problems.
  d. guides the nurse to record important information.

2. Continuity of care is demonstrated in POMR charting because:
  a. a continuous chronologic list of problems is made.
  b. the priority of problems is identified by numbering them.
  c. the plan of care and interventions are recorded together.
  d. an initial list of problems is the one followed for continuing care.

3. In PIE charting, the P stands for:
  a. plan.
  b. problem.
  c. practice.
  d. progress.

4. In focus charting, DAR stands for:
  a. data, action, response.
  b. date, activity, revision.

    c. date, assessment, record.
    d. data, activity, requirements.

5. Computerized charting:
    a. reduces accuracy.
    b. decreases legibility.
    c. ensures everything is confidential.
    d. follows the components of the nursing process.

Critical Thinking Questions

1. How could the problems with computerized charting be overcome?

2. Why are there so many methods of documentation? Of what value is each?

WEB FLASH!

- Check the Internet for information on each of the methods of documentation. What additional material do you find?
- Go to www.about.com to see what is available about documentation.

References/Suggested Readings

Aquilino, M., & Keenan, G. (2000). Having our say: Nursing's standardized nomenclature. *AJN, 100*(7), 33–38.

Beyea, S. (1996). *Critical pathways for collaborative nursing care.* Menlo Park, CA: Addison-Wesley Nursing.

Burke, L. J., & Murphy, J. (1995). *Charting by exception applications.* Albany, NY: Delmar.

Charting Tips. (1999a). Documenting discharges and transfers in long-term care. *Nursing99, 29*(6), 17.

Charting Tips. (1999b). Easy as PIE. *Nursing99, 29*(4), 24.

DeWitt, A. (2000). *Documentation: Legal principles of good charting.* Penumbra Seminars LLC [On-line]. Available: www.respiratorycare-online.com/doc_handout.pdf

Dumpel, H., James, M., and Phillips, T. (1999). Charting by exception. *California Nurse*, June/July 1999, p. 9 Also [On-line]. Available: www.califnurses.org/cna/cal/junju99/9cnjj99.html

Dykes, P., and Wheeler, K. (Eds.) (1997). *Planning, implementing and evaluating critical pathways*. New York: Springer.

Eggland, E. T., & Heinemann, D. S. (1994). *Nursing documentation: Charting, recording, and reporting*. Philadelphia: Lippincott Williams & Wilkins.

Fiesta, J. (1991). If it wasn't charted, it was done! *Nursing Management*, 22(8), 17.

Grulke, C. C. (1995). Seven ways to help a student nurse. *AJN*, 96(60), 24L.

Habel, M. (2000a). *Documenting patient care, Part 1* [On-line]. Available: www.nurseweek.com/ce/ce10a.html

Habel, M. (2000b). *Documenting patient care Part 2* [On-line]. Available: www.nurseweek.com/ce/ce20a.html

Iowa Interventions Project. (1993). The NIC taxonomy structure. *Image: Journal of Nursing Scholarship, 25*(3), 187–192.

Iyer, P. W., & Camp, N. H. (1999). *Nursing documentation: A nursing process approach* (3rd ed.). St. Louis, MO: Mosby.

Joint Commission on Accreditation of Healthcare Organizations. (1998). *1998 Hospital accreditation standards*. Oakbrook Terrace, IL: Author.

Klenner, S. (2000). Mapping out a clinical pathway, *RN, 63*(6), 33–36.

Pethtel, P. (2000). *Nursing documentation*. [On-line] Available: http://garnet.indstate.edu/ppethtel/chartingforweb/

Rochman, R. (2000). Are computerized patient records for you? *Nursing2000, 30*(10), 61–62.

Smith, L. (2000a). How to use focus charting. *Nursing2000, 30*(5), 76.

Smith, L. (2000b). Safe computer charting. *Nursing2000, 30*(9), 85.

Springhouse. (1999). *Mastering documentation* (2nd ed.). Springhouse, PA: Author.

Sullivan, G. (2000). Keep your charting on course. *RN, 63*(5), 75–79.

Thede, L. (1999). *Computers in nursing: Bridges to the future*. Philadelphia, PA: Lippincott Williams & Wilkins.

Thompson, C. (1995). Writing better narrative notes. *Nursing95, 25*(5), 87.

White, L. (2001). *Foundations of nursing: Caring for the whole person*. Albany, NY: Delmar.

White, L. (2002). *Basic nursing: Foundations of skills & concepts*. Albany, NY: Delmar.

RESOURCES

American Nursing Informatics Association (ANIA). PMB105, 10808 Foothill Boulevard, Suite 160, Rancho Cucamonga, CA 91730, http://www.ania.org

Center for Nursing Classification, The University of Iowa, College of Nursing, 407 Nursing Building, Iowa City, IA 52242-1121, 319-335-7051, http://www.nursing.uiowa.edu

Medical Records Institute, P.O. Box 600770, 567 Walnut Street, Newton, MA 02460, 617-964-3923, www.medrecinst.com

North American Nursing Diagnosis Association (NANDA). 1211 Locust Street, Philadelphia, PA 19107, 800-647-9002, http://www.nanda.org

CHAPTER
10

FORMS FOR RECORDING DATA

INTRODUCTION

There are several types of forms on which nurses record data about a client: Kardex, flow sheets, nurses' progress notes, and discharge summaries. All these forms are designed to facilitate record keeping, minimize duplication of effort, and ensure quick and easy access to information.

KARDEX

A **Kardex** is a summary worksheet reference of basic client care information traditionally not part of the medical record (Figure 10-1). A concise client data source, Kardex is used as a reference throughout the shift and during change-of-shift reports. Kardexes come in various sizes, shapes, and types, including computer-generated. The Kardex is designed to assist those working in the care delivery setting and usually contains the following information:

- Client data: name, age, marital status, religious preference, physician, family contact with phone number
- Medical diagnoses: listed by priority
- Nursing diagnoses: listed by priority
- Allergies
- Medical orders: diet, medications, intravenous (IV) therapy, treatments, diagnostic tests and procedures (inclusive of dates and results), consultations, DNR (do-not-resuscitate) order (when appropriate)
- Activities permitted: functional limitations, assistance needed in activities of daily living, and safety precautions

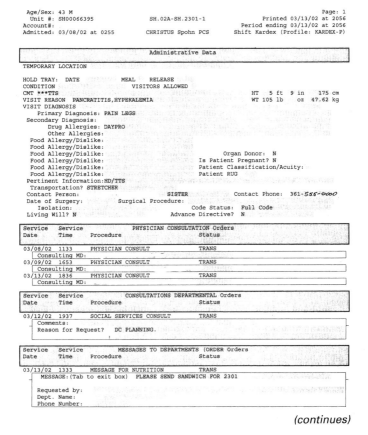

```
Age/Sex:  43 M                                                      Page: 1
  Unit #: SH00066395           SH.02A-SH.2301-1       Printed 03/13/02 at 2056
Account#:                                             Period ending 03/13/02 at 2056
Admitted:  03/08/02 at 0255     CHRISTUS Spohn PCS    Shift Kardex (Profile: KARDEX-P)
```

```
                            Administrative Data

TEMPORARY LOCATION

HOLD TRAY:  DATE          MEAL     RELEASE
CONDITION                 VISITORS ALLOWED
CMT ***TTS                                            HT    5 ft   9 in    175 cm
VISIT REASON   PANCRATITIS,HYPEKALEMIA                WT 105 lb    oz   47.62 kg
VISIT DIAGNOSIS
   Primary Diagnosis:  PAIN LEGS
Secondary Diagnosis:
   Drug Allergies:  DAYPRO
   Other Allergies:
Food Allergy/Dislike:
Food Allergy/Dislike:
Food Allergy/Dislike:                                 Organ Donor:  N
Food Allergy/Dislike:                    Is Patient Pregnant? N
Food Allergy/Dislike:                    Patient Classification/Acuity:
Food Allergy/Dislike:                    Patient RUG
Pertinent Information:HD/TTS
Transportation? STRETCHER
Contact Person:                   SISTER          Contact Phone:  361-555-0000
Date of Surgery:           Surgical Procedure:
   Isolation:                            Code Status:  Full Code
Living Will? N                          Advance Directive?  N
```

Service Date	Service Time	Procedure	PHYSICIAN CONSULTATION Orders	Status
03/08/02	1133	PHYSICIAN CONSULT		TRANS
		Consulting MD:		
03/09/02	1653	PHYSICIAN CONSULT		TRANS
		Consulting MD:		
03/13/02	1836	PHYSICIAN CONSULT		TRANS
		Consulting MD:		

Service Date	Service Time	Procedure	CONSULTATIONS DEPARTMENTAL Orders	Status
03/12/02	1937	SOCIAL SERVICES CONSULT		TRANS
		Comments:		
		Reason for Request? DC PLANNING.		

Service Date	Service Time	Procedure	MESSAGES TO DEPARTMENTS (ORDER Orders	Status
03/13/02	1333	MESSAGE FOR NUTRITION		TRANS
		MESSAGE:(Tab to exit box) PLEASE SEND SANDWICH FOR 2301		
		Requested by:		
		Dept. Name:		
		Phone Number:		

(continues)

Figure 10-1 Example of Kardex (Courtesy of CHRISTUS Spohn Health System, Corpus Christi, TX)

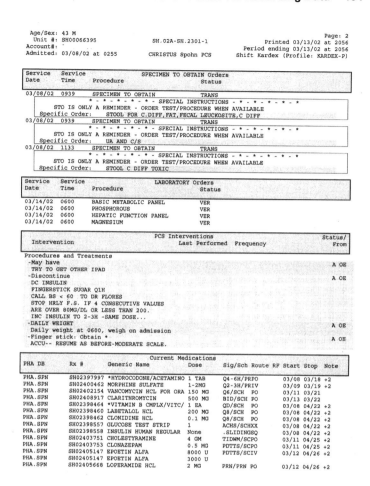

Figure 10-1 *(continued)*

FLOW SHEETS

Flow sheets have columns for recording dates and times for assessments and/or intervention information, making it easy to track changes in the client's condition. Client teaching, use of special equipment, and IV therapy may also be included in a flow sheet. Because flow sheets have small spaces for recording, these forms usually contain legends that identify the approved abbreviations for charting data (Figure 10-2). It is important to fill out flow sheets completely because blank spaces imply that an assessment or intervention was not completed, attempted, or recognized.

Date:

Nutrition:	Hygiene:	7-3	3-11	11-7
Diet □ NPO □	Bath □ Sitz □	self □ assist □ total	self □ assist □ total	self □ assist □ total
Hyperal □ Tube Fed □	Shower □	refused □	refused □	refused □
Breakfast:	Oral Care	self □	assist □	Total	self □	assist □	Total	self □	assist □	Total
All >½ <½ 0	Shave	self □	assist □	Total	self □	assist □	Total	self □	assist □	Total
□ □ □ □	Peri Care	self □	assist □	Total	self □	assist □	Total	self □	assist □	Total
Lunch:	Other:			
All >½ <½ 0				
□ □ □ □	Comments:			
Dinner:				
All >½ <½ 0				
□ □ □ □				
Snacks:				
All >½ <½ 0				
□ □ □ □				

Tube Feeding Residuals				Intake					Output			
Time	Amount	7-3	PO	IV	NG & Flush	Enteral	Other	Urine	Ng/Emesis	Stool	Drains
		7-3 Total									
Weight		3-11									
Today:											
Previous:											
Vital/Signs											
Time T P R B/P P/S		3-11 Total									
		11-7									
		11-7 Total									
		24° / Total									

CHRISTUS SPOHN HEALTH SYSTEM

FLOW SHEET - 24 HOUR RECORD
PATIENT CARE SERVICES
2705066

4010

REV. 06/00

(continues)

Figure 10-2 Example of Flow Sheet—24 Hour Record (Courtesy of CHRISTUS Spohn Health System, Corpus Christi, TX)

Because they decrease the redundancy of charting in the nurses' progress notes, flow sheets are used as supplements to most documentation systems. They do not, however, replace the progress notes. Nurses still must document observations, client responses and teaching, detailed interventions, and other significant data in the progress notes.

	Date:	7-3 Time:	3-11 Time:	11-7 Time:
Neuro	Normal: alert, oriented to time, place, person, follows command, speech clear	WNL: ☐ *	WNL: ☐ *	WNL: ☐ *
Respira-tory	Normal: Regular, unlabored symmetrical respirations, no abnormal lung sounds	WNL: ☐ *	WNL: ☐ *	WNL: ☐ *
Cardio-vascular	Normal: Heart rhythm regular, peripheral pulses easily palpable and strong bilaterally, no edema, capillary refill brisk	WNL: ☐ *	WNL: ☐ *	WNL: ☐ *
Musculo-Skeletal	Normal: Full ROM of All joints, no weakness, steady balance and gait, handgrips equal	WNL: ☐ *	WNL: ☐ *	WNL: ☐ *
Nutrition	Normal: Consumes greater than 1/2 of solid food meals	WNL: ☐ *	WNL: ☐ *	WNL: ☐ *
G.I.	Normal: Abdomen soft, bowel sounds present all 4 quadrants, no nausea/ vomiting, diarrhea/constipation Last BM:	WNL: ☐ *	WNL: ☐ *	WNL: ☐ *
G.U.	Normal: Voiding without difficulty, clear urine, no bladder distention	WNL: ☐ *	WNL: ☐ *	WNL: ☐ *
Skin	Normal: Skin warm, dry, intact, tugor elastic, oral cavity moist and intact Date of Last EZ Graph _____ Site: _____	WNL: ☐ *	WNL: ☐ *	WNL: ☐ *
Psycho-social	Normal: Thought processes logical, memory intact, behavior appropriate for situation	WNL: ☐ *	WNL: ☐ *	WNL: ☐ *
Incision	Normal: Incision clean, no redness, drainage Site: _____	WNL: ☐ *	WNL: ☐ *	WNL: ☐ *
Wound	Normal: Dry, no drainage, no odor Site: _____	WNL: ☐ *	WNL: ☐ *	WNL: ☐ *

Safety Assess-ment	STATUS: MENTAL/PHYSICAL	MEDICATIONS	HISTORY
	D E N ☐☐☐ (5) Confused/judgement impaired ☐☐☐ (5) Sensory impairment ☐☐☐ (5) Combative/aggressive ☐☐☐ (5) "Sundowners" syndrome ☐☐☐ (5) Noncompliance/uncooperative ☐☐☐ (5) Paralysis/amputee ☐☐☐ (5) Urgent/frequent elimination needs ☐☐☐ (10) Restraints in use ☐☐☐ (5) Weakness/debilitation/mobility impaired TOTAL D _____	D E N ☐☐☐ (5) Diuretics ☐☐☐ (5) Laxatives/G.I. preps ☐☐☐ (3) Antihypertensives ☐☐☐ (3) Antiseizures ☐☐☐ (5) Sedative/hypnotics ☐☐☐ (3) Analgesics ☐☐☐ (3) Antipsychotics/ antidepressants E _____	D E N ☐☐☐ (5) Age greater than 60 ☐☐☐ (5) History of previous falls ☐☐☐ (3) From nursing home ☐☐☐ (3) Has had sitter/ companion at home SAFETY LEVEL D E N ☐☐☐ Level 1 (0-17) ☐☐☐ Level 2 (18-24) ☐☐☐ Level 3 (25 or greater) N _____

(continues)

Figure 10-2 *(continued)*

COMMUNITY/HOME HEALTH CARE

Home Health Kardex

In addition to the usual information, the home health Kardex contains information related to family contacts, practitioners (physician), other services, and emergency referrals.

		EDUCATION REASSESSMENT

Have the Education needs of the patient changed in past 24 hours?   ☐ Yes   ☐ No
Is the patient scheduled for any new test or procedure today?   ☐ Yes   ☐ No
Explanation given?   ☐ Yes   ☐ No
Patient/significant other verbalizes understanding: ☐ Yes   ☐ No
Patient desires/requires education on: _____

Have Discharge Planning needs changed in past 24 hours?   ☐ Yes   ☐ No
If yes, send consult to Social Services and document changes below.

ALL EDUCATION MUST BE DOCUMENTED ON THE MULTIDISCIPLINARY EDUCATION FORM

TIME	PROBLEM #	PROGRESS NOTES

(continues)

Figure 10-2 *(continued)*

NURSES' PROGRESS NOTES

Nurses' progress notes are used to document the client's condition, problems, and complaints; interventions; the client's response to interventions; and achievement of outcomes. Progress notes can be either completely narrative or incorporated into a standardized flow sheet to complement SOAP(IE), PIE, focus charting, and other documentation systems.

TIME	PROBLEM #	PROGRESS NOTES

PLAN OF CARE VERIFICATION _____ RN _____ Time

IV SITE ASSESSMENT		7-3 Time:	3-11 Time:	11-7 Time:
Normal: IV Patent; No redness, drainage or edema	Site #1: Start Date:	WNL: ☐ *	WNL: ☐ *	WNL: ☐ *
# of IVAC's in use ___	Site #2: Start Date:	WNL: ☐ *	WNL: ☐ *	WNL: ☐ *
IV Site Care per hospital standard ☐ Time:			*	
IV Tubing Change per hospital standard ☐ Time:			*	

IV Start:	Time	Attempts	Site	Needle Size	S	U
					☐	☐
Site prep per Standard ☐					☐	☐
					☐	☐

INITIALS	SIGNATURE	INITIALS	SIGNATURE

Figure 10-2 *(continued)*

Forms that come under the general heading of nurses' progress notes include: Personal Care Flow Sheet (Figure 10-2) that includes Nurses' Progress Notes on pages 3 and 4 and Intake & Output Record on page 1, MAR (Figure 10-3), Teaching Record (Figure 10-4), and specialty forms such as Diabetic Flow Sheet (Figure 10-5) and Neurologic Assessment Form (Figure 10-6).

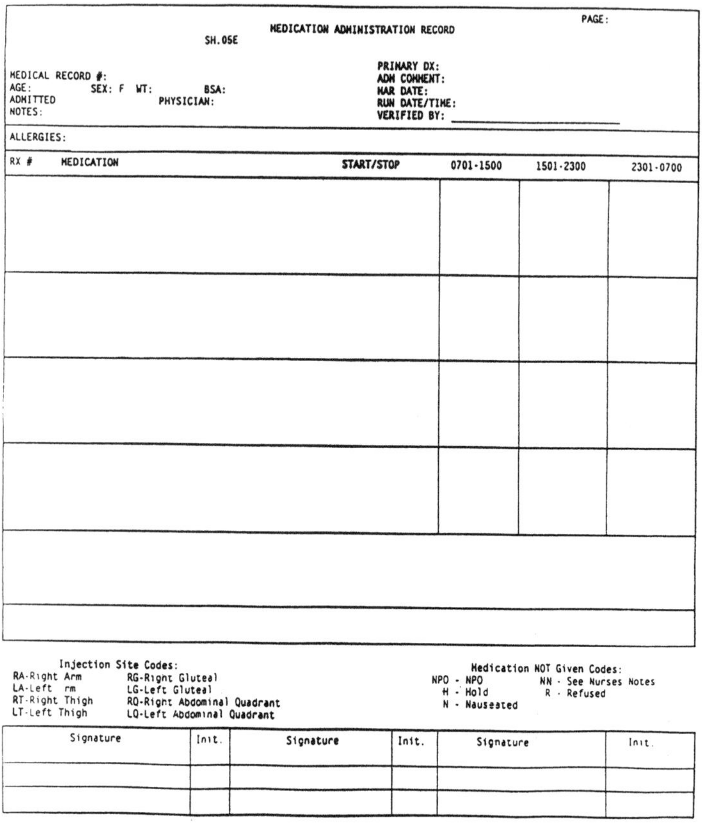

MEDICATION ADMINISTRATION RECORD
SH.05E
PAGE:

MEDICAL RECORD #:
AGE: SEX: F WT: BSA:
ADMITTED PHYSICIAN:
NOTES:

PRIMARY DX:
ADM COMMENT:
MAR DATE:
RUN DATE/TIME:
VERIFIED BY:

ALLERGIES:

RX # MEDICATION START/STOP	0701-1500	1501-2300	2301-0700

Injection Site Codes:
RA-Right Arm, RG-Right Gluteal
LA-Left rm, LG-Left Gluteal
RT-Right Thigh, RQ-Right Abdominal Quadrant
LT-Left Thigh, LQ-Left Abdominal Quadrant

Medication NOT Given Codes:
NPO - NPO, NN - See Nurses Notes
H - Hold, R - Refused
N - Nauseated

Signature	Init.	Signature	Init.	Signature	Init.

Figure 10-3 Example of MAR (medication administration record) (Courtesy of CHRISTUS Spohn Health System, Corpus Christi, TX)

DISCHARGE SUMMARY

The discharge summary highlights the client's illness and course of care. When a narrative discharge summary is entered into the progress notes, it includes:

- The client's status at admission and discharge;
- A brief summary of the client's care;

INITIAL EDUCATIONAL ASSESSMENT

EDUCATIONAL
Patient Family Learning Needs: (initial all that apply:)
__ Present Illness   __ Rehabilitation __ Hypertension   __ Diabetes   __ Heart Disease __ Cancer
__ Incontinence   __ Medications   __ Diet   __ Skin Care   __ Post-Op Care   __ Home Equipment
__ Community resources   __ Personal hygiene & grooming   __ * Other _____

All "yes" answers require comment   Patient/Family Ability to Learn:
*Physical Limitations: ___ No ___ Yes   *Cognitive Limitations: ___ No ___ Yes   *Emotional Barriers: ___ No ___ Yes
*Language Barrier: ___ No ___ Yes   *Primary Language Spoken ___ English ___ Spanish ___ Other: _____
                                         Ability to read ___ English ___ Spanish ___ Other ___ None
Religious or cultural practices that may impact care of education ___ No ___ Yes   Age Considerations ___ No ___ Yes
Financial implications of care choices. ___ No ___ Yes   (Reference Milestones Growth and Development Guide)
COMMENTS: _____
Patient/Family Preferences for Learning: (Initial all that apply:)
___ Video   ___ Demonstration   ___ 1 to 1 instruction   ___ Handout material
___ Other (please comment) _____
Patient/Family Readiness to Learn: ___ Express readiness ___ Express desire to delay learning (Comment) _____
Date: _____ Time: _____ Signature: _____

KEYS:
Learner	Teaching Methods	Limitations to Learning	Evaluation	
Patient [P] Spouse [S]	Written Material [W] Video [V]	None [1] Pain [2] Anxiety [3]	States Understanding	[S]
Family [F] Other [O]	Demonstration [D] Explanation [E]	Physical Limitation [4]	Reference (See CPG,	
Demonstration [D]		Unable to Understand [5]	Problem List Teaching Records)	[Ref]
Video [V]		Disinterested [6]	No Indication Learning Has Occurred	[N]
			Return Demonstration	[R]
			Needs ongoing instruction [O]	

DATE	TIME	CONTENT	LEARNER	TEACHING METHODS	LIMITA TIONS	EVALUA TION	SIGNATURE/ DEPT.
		Discussion of disease process, diagnosis, or condition.(Specify)_____					
		Signs and Symptoms Risk Factors					
		Treatment Modalities					
		Follow-up Care _____					
		Pre Op Teaching/Preparation for diagnostic tests/invasive procedure (Specify)_____					
		Post Op Teaching for invasive procedures (Specify)_____					
		Food/Drug interactions (list drugs)					
		Diet Education					
		Medication Use (List drugs)					
		Medical Equipment (List)					
		No Need Identified					
		CHRISTUS SPOHN HEALTH SYSTEM MULTIDISCIPLINARY EDUCATION RECORD PATIENT CARE SERVICES 2705187 NEW: 07/99 REVISED: 06/04/2001 FM 15					
		Rehabilitation (Describe)					

(continues)

Figure 10-4 Example of Teaching Record (Courtesy of CHRISTUS Spohn Health System, Corpus Christi, TX)

- Intervention and education outcomes;
- Resolved problems and continuing care needs for unresolved problems, inclusive of referrals; and
- Client instructions regarding medications, diet, food–drug interactions, activity, treatments, follow-up, and other special needs.

DATE	TIME	CONTENT	LEARNER	TEACHING METHODS	LIMITATIONS	EVALUATION	SIGNATURE/ DEPT.
		PT _____ TR _____ OT _____ Speech _____					
		Special Treatments (Describe)					
		Community Resources (Specify) _____					
		Discharge Planning [ ] Condition that may result in transfer [ ] Alternative to transfer [ ] Clinical basis and time frame for D/C [ ] Need for continued care at D/C					
		Diabetes Teaching [ ] DM Medication [ ] Insulin Adm. Techniques [ ] Diet Guidelines [ ] Hypoglycemia – Sx., Tx, Prev. [ ] Foot Care [ ] Sick Day Guidelines [ ] Blood Glucose Monitoring					
		Explanation of safety program, level precautions, and wristband					
		Topic: Pain Management Information and Education					
		Topic _____					
		Topic _____					
		Topic _____					
		Topic _____					
		Topic _____					
		Topic _____					
		Topic _____					
		Topic _____					
		Topic _____					

05/30/01   FM15

Figure 10-4 *(continued)*

Many facilities have a documentation form that itemizes discharge and client instructions. The form has a duplicate copy for the client, with the original being placed in the medical record. Figure 10-7 shows the common elements of this tool.

SUMMARY

- Many forms are used by nurses to record data about a client; these forms may also vary from facility to facility.
- A Kardex is a summary worksheet reference not generally part of the medical record.

INITIAL / SIGNATURE:		INJECTION SITE:	INSULIN:

INITIAL / SIGNATURE:

1.___/___   5.___/___
2.___/___   6.___/___
3.___/___   7.___/___
4.___/___   8.___/___

INJECTION SITE:
RA - Right Arm
LA - Left Arm
RT - Right Thigh
LT - Left Thigh
RUQ – Right Upper Abdominal Quadrant
LUQ – Left Upper Abdominal Quadrant
RLQ – Right Lower Abdominal Quadrant
LLQ – Left Lower Abdominal Quadrant

INSULIN:
H – HUMALOG/NOVOLOG
R – REGULAR
N – NPH
L – LENTE
U – ULTRA LENTE
G - GLARGINE
M - 70/30
P - 75/25
A - Alternative

DATE		0400-0759	0800-1159	1200-1559	1600-1959	2000-2359	2400-0359	TOTAL DAILY DOSE	HYPO/ HYPERGLYCEMIA INTERVENTIONS			INT
	Time of B.S.								DATE/TIME	B.S.	TREATMENT	
	Blood Glucose											
	Time of Sliding Scale Insulin											
	Sliding Scale Dose											
	Injection Site/Initial											
	Time of Insulin											
	Insulin Scheduled Dose											
	Injection Site/Initial											
	Time of B.S.											
	Blood Glucose											
	Time of Sliding Scale Insulin											
	Sliding Scale Dose											
	Injection Site/Initial											
	Time of Insulin											
	Insulin Scheduled Dose											
	Injection Site/Initial											
	Time of B.S.											
	Blood Glucose											
	Time of Sliding Scale Insulin											
	Sliding Scale Dose											
	Injection Site/Initial											
	Time of Insulin											
	Insulin Scheduled Dose											
	Injection Site/Initial											

CHRISTUS SPOHN HEALTH SYSTEM

DIABETES BLOOD GLUCOSE / INSULIN ADMINISTRATION
FLOWSHEET- PATIENT CARE SERVICES

2006
2704946   NEW: 2/2001
                NSAFM12

Figure 10-5 Example of Diabetic Flow Sheet (Courtesy of CHRISTUS Spohn Health System, Corpus Christi, TX)

- Flow sheets make it easy to track changes in the client's condition.
- The discharge summary highlights the client's illness and course of care.

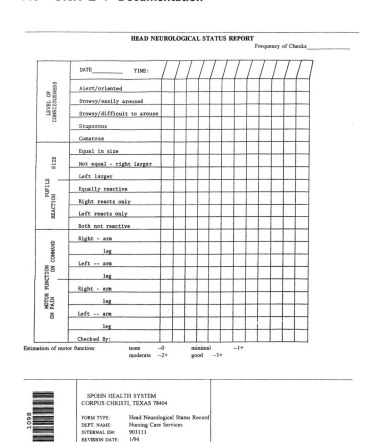

Figure 10-6 Example of Neurologic Assessment Form (Courtesy of CHRISTUS Spohn Health System, Corpus Christi, TX)

Review Questions

1. The Kardex is used as:
  a. a reference.
  b. a record of all client care.
  c. the second sheet of a client record.
  d. the place for physicians to write orders.

Follow-up: To be seen in _____ office on _____
              (Dr. Name/Clinic)   (date/time)

Follow-up: To be seen in _____ office on _____
              (Dr. Name/Clinic)   (date/time)

Follow-up: To be seen in _____ office on _____
              (Dr. Name/Clinic)   (date/time)

DIET: _____ Diet instruction given to patient _____
                                       (Period of time/date)

ACTIVITY_____ Services: ○ Home Health ○ Hospice ○ DME

Treatments/Self Care _____ Other (Specify): _____

Drug Nutrient Interactions _____ Return to: _____ for

○ PT ○ OT ○ RT ○ Other _____

MEDICATIONS	DOSAGE	FREQUENCY	MEDICATIONS	DOSAGE	FREQUENCY

MEDICATION CONTROL INSTRUCTIONS:
1. Take your medication according to M.D. instructions.
2. Never stop taking your medication without speaking to your M.D.
3. Refill your medication when you have 7 days worth left.
4. Notify your M.D. if your pain medication needs adjusting; you are having uncontrolled pain or you are having difficulty with side effects.

_____ Preprinted Instructions Given to Patient/Family   Other Instructions: _____

CHRISTUS Spohn associates trust we have met your needs while in the hospital. Shortly after discharge, you will receive a patient survey. It is our hope that you will circle high scores of 5s when you take a few moments to complete and mail the survey. I understand and am able to implement continuing care needs at home as explained to me.

_____ (Patient/Family Signature)

Admission Date _____ Discharge Date _____ Via: _____ Escorted by: _____
                                       Time: _____ Destination: _____

PATIENT DISCHARGE STATUS

1. Vital Signs _____
2. Elimination-Date of last BM _____
   GU _____
3. Neuro _____
4. Cardiac _____

5. Resp _____
6. Skin/Wound/Incisions _____
7. Vascular Access Removed _____
8. Pain Free: No But Controlled by Pain Medication
             Yes, at time of Discharge _____

9. Other _____

	Yes	No	N/A
Own medications from home returned to patient/family.	_____	_____	_____
Prescriptions given to patient/family.	_____	_____	_____
Valuables returned to patient/family.	_____	_____	_____

Original to chart, copy to Patient/Family

Signature/Title Discharge Nurse: _____ Date: _____

CHRISTUS Spohn Health System

DISCHARGE INFORMATION RECORD
PATIENT CARE SERVICES

1045

2704965   REV: 05/00 FM7

Figure 10-7 Example of Discharge Summary (Courtesy of CHRISTUS Spohn Health System, Corpus Christi, TX)

2. Flow sheets:
   a. are a documentation system.
   b. replace nurses progress notes.
   c. are only used in postoperative situation.
   d. make it easy to track changes in a client's condition.

3. Forms that fall under the general heading of nurse's progress notes include:
   a. personal care flow sheet, MAR, and I&O form.
   b. MAR, teaching records, and discharge summary.
   c. I&O forms, nurses notes, and admission assessment.
   d. admission assessment, personal care flow sheet, and discharge summary.

4. The discharge summary:
   a. is only for the client.
   b. itemizes client instructions.
   c. is not part of the client's record.
   d. details client care and education outcomes.

Critical Thinking Questions

1. How do flow sheets complement a client's record?

2. Why is the discharge summary important to the client? To the physician? To the health care facility?

WEB FLASH!

- What can you find on the Internet about the various methods of charting?
- Search the Internet for information about NIC and NOC. How can you use this information?

References/Suggested Readings

Fiesta, J. (1991). If it wasn't charted, it was done! *Nursing Management, 22*(8), 17.

Gardner, P. (2002). *Nursing process in action.* Albany, NY: Delmar.

Joint Commission on Accreditation of Healthcare Organizations. (1998). *1998 Hospital accreditation standards.* Oakbrook Terrace, IL: Author.

Seaback, W. (2001). *Nursing process: Concepts & application.* Albany, NY: Delmar.

Springhouse. (1999). *Mastering documentation* (2nd ed.). Springhouse, PA: Author.

White, L. (2001). *Foundations of nursing: Caring for the whole person.* Albany, NY: Delmar.

White, L. (2002). *Basic nursing: Foundations of skills & concepts.* Albany, NY: Delmar.

CHAPTER 11

TRENDS IN DOCUMENTATION

LEARNING OBJECTIVES

Upon completion of this chapter, you should be able to:
- *Define key terms.*
- *Discuss the following trends in documentation: nursing minimum data set, nursing diagnosis, nursing interventions classification, and nursing outcomes classification.*

KEY TERMS

Nursing Interventions
  Classification
nursing minimum data set

Nursing Outcomes
  Classification

INTRODUCTION

Computerized charting has become one of the most widespread trends in nursing documentation. However, computerized nursing documentation can demonstrate the quality, effectiveness, and value of the services nurses provide only if standardized databases are developed that will ensure accuracy and precision in the information. At the 1991 conference of the National Center for Nursing Research of the National Institutes of Health, the need was identified for databases that would permit analysis of the effectiveness and costs of specific interventions in achieving desired outcomes for clients with a variety of nursing diagnoses (Ozbolt, Fruchtnight, & Hayden, 1994). The recommendations arising from this conference supported the need to define and develop standard terminology for nursing data, nursing diagnoses, nursing interventions, and nursing outcomes.

NURSING MINIMUM DATA SET

In 1985, Werley and Lang convened an invitational working conference at the University of Wisconsin–Milwaukee to identify the elements that should be included in a **nursing minimum data set** (NMDS). These are the elements that they felt should be contained in client records which could then be abstracted for studies on the effectiveness and costs of nursing care (Werley & Lang, 1988). The sixteen identified elements were grouped into the following three categories:

* Demographics: personal identification, date of birth, gender, race and ethnicity, and residence
* Service: unique facility or service agency number, episode admission or encounter date, discharge or termination date, disposition of client, expected payer, unique health record number of client, and unique number of principal registered nurse provider
* Nursing care: nursing diagnosis, nursing intervention, nursing outcome, and intensity of nursing care (Werley & Lang, 1988)

Several challenges are inherent in the development of the four nursing care categories: diagnoses, interventions, outcomes, and intensity (Hayes et al., 1994). For example, automated information systems must be capable of supporting cost-effective nursing practice through efficient, comprehensive documentation. Further, basic to standardizing databases is the consistent use of a taxonomy that promotes validity and reliability. The NMDS, however, does not specify for any of the four elements under nursing care a taxonomy such as NANDA (2001) nursing diagnoses, Nursing Interventions Classification (NIC) (NIC, 1995), Nursing Outcomes Classification (NOC), or acuity ratings. Nursing must achieve consensus of terminology in order for clinical data to be included in nursing care elements of a NMDS.

NURSING DIAGNOSES

The North American Nursing Diagnosis Association (NANDA) is recognized as the pioneer in diagnostic classification in nursing. The NANDA definition of a nursing diagnosis is: "A nursing diagnosis is a clinical judgment about individual, family, or community responses to actual or potential health problems or life processes" (NANDA, 2001). Currently, there are 155 approved nursing diagnoses classified into 13 domains. The thirteen domains are:

- Health Promotion
- Nutrition
- Elimination
- Activity/Rest
- Perception/Cognition
- Self-Perception
- Role Relationships
- Sexuality
- Coping/Stress Tolerance
- Life Principles
- Safety/Protection
- Comfort
- Growth/Development

Many diagnostic labels (nursing diagnoses) now have new descriptors. The word "altered" has been removed and a more specific term used. This allows for more specific documentation and for the nursing diagnoses to be linked to NIC and NOC. The nursing diagnoses are listed in alphabetical order by the diagnostic concept not by the first word of the nursing diagnosis (NANDA, 2001). For example: *Excess Fluid Volume* is found under "fluid." The entire listing can be found in Appendix A. Each diagnosis has a label, definition, defining characteristics, and related factors. The diagnoses identify client states which can then be used to select interventions that are intended to achieve desired outcomes.

In 1992, the NANDA terms were accepted into the Unified Medical Language System (UMLS). The UMLS was begun in 1986 by the National Library of Medicine as a way to help health professionals and researchers retrieve and integrate electronic biomedical information from a variety of sources (National Library of Medicine, 2000).

NURSING INTERVENTIONS CLASSIFICATION

The **Nursing Interventions Classification** (NIC) is a comprehensive standardized classification of nursing interventions organized in a three-level taxonomy. This taxonomy sorts, labels, and describes interventions used by nurses for various diagnostic categories. Initiated by a research team (Iowa Intervention Project, 1993) at the University of Iowa in 1987, the three-level taxonomy now comprises 7 domains, 30 classes, and almost 500 interventions. The seven domains are:

- Physiological: basic
- Physiological: complex
- Behavioral
- Safety
- Family
- Health system
- Community

A nursing intervention is any direct care treatment that a nurse performs on behalf of a client (Gordon, 1998). These treatments include nurse-initiated treatments resulting from nursing diagnoses, physician-initiated treatments resulting from medical diagnoses, and performance of the daily essential functions for the client who cannot do these.

Each nursing intervention has four parts: the intervention label, the intervention definition, a set of activities to carry out the interventions, and a list of references. *Activities are not interventions and should not be labeled as such in nursing information systems* (McCloskey & Bulechek, 2000).

The strengths of the Nursing Interventions Classification include the following:

- Comprehensive—includes full range of nursing interventions; can be used in any practice setting.
- Researched Based—research used a multimethod approach.
- Reflects Current Clinical Practice—all interventions reviewed by experts in clinical practice; each intervention has a list of references.
- Has Easy to Use Organizing Structure—all domains, classes, and interventions have definitions; interventions are numerically coded.
- Uses Language That Is Clear and Clinically Meaningful—language most useful in clinical practice was selected.
- Linked to NANDA Nursing Diagnoses and NOC Client Outcomes—linkage lists are available (The University of Iowa College of Nursing, 2001a).

COMMUNITY/HOME HEALTH CARE

Taxonomy of Nursing Interventions
Grobe and colleagues at the University of Texas at Austin have been developing a lexicon and taxonomy of nursing interventions taken from home care records (Grobe, 1992).

While continuing to evolve, this classification system provides assistance in choosing interventions based on nursing diagnoses or problems. The NIC interventions have been incorporated into health care data sets and the computerized client medical record. The ANA has recognized NIC as one of the first nursing languages to be included in the *National Library of Medicine's Metathesaurus,* one of four knowledge sources for the UMLS.

NURSING OUTCOMES CLASSIFICATION

An outcome is a measurable individual, family, or community state, behavior or perception that is measured along a continuum and is responsive to nursing interventions (The University of Iowa College of Nursing, 2001b).

The Iowa Outcomes Project being conducted at the University of Iowa has developed a taxonomy of client outcomes for nursing care, using comprehensive standardized language called **Nursing Outcomes Classification** (NOC). This classification of client outcomes was developed to evaluate the effects of nursing interventions. It comprises 260 outcomes grouped into 29 classes and 7 domains (Johnson, Maas, & Moorhead, 2000).

The seven domains are:

- Functional health
- Physiologic health
- Psychosocial health
- Health knowledge and behavior

- Perceived health
- Family health
- Community health

Each NOC outcome has five parts: the outcome label, the outcome definition, a list of indicators for measurement, a five-point measurement scale, and a list of references (Aquilino & Keenan, 2000). The ANA has recognized NOC as a standardized language and it is included in the *National Library of Medicine's Metathesaurus* for a Unified Medical Language (NCVHS, 1999).

SUMMARY

- Computerized charting has become one of the most widespread trends in nursing documentation.
- Nursing minimum data set identifies elements that should be in a clinical record which can then be abstracted for studies on the effectiveness and costs of nursing care.
- NANDA nursing diagnoses identify client states that can be used to select interventions intended to achieve desired outcomes.
- NIC sorts, labels, and describes nursing interventions.
- NOC defines outcomes, lists indicators for measurement, and provides a measurement scale.
- NANDA, NIC, and NOC are now linked together.

Review Questions

1. One of the most widespread trends in nursing documentation is:
   a. charting by exception.
   b. computerized charting.
   c. accuracy and precision in information records.
   d. demonstrating quality and effectiveness of nursing services.

2. Each nursing intervention in (NIC) has:
   a. indicators and activities.
   b. a label and a measurement scale.
   c. a label, a definition, and activities.
   d. a definition, indicators, and references.

3. The NOC nursing outcomes were developed to:
   a. identify community needs.
   b. define how clients should respond.
   c. measure individual or family behavior.
   d. evaluate the effects of nursing interventions.

Critical Thinking Questions

1. Why is a nursing minimum data set important?

2. Compare NANDA, NIC, and NOC.

WEB FLASH!

- Search the web for current developments in: NIC, NOC, and NMDS.
- Go to the NANDA web site at www.nanda.org to find the latest developments about nursing diagnoses.

References/Suggested Readings

Aquilino, M., & Keenan, G. (2000). Having our say: Nursing's standardized nomenclature, *AJN, 100*(7), 33–38.

Clark, M. (1998). Implementation of nursing standardized languages. NANDA, NIC, and NOC. *On-line Journal of Issues in Nursing, 2*(2) [On-line]. Available: http://www.nursingworld.org

Daly, J., Button, P., Prophet, C., Clarke, M., & Androwich, I. (1997). Nursing interventions classification implementation issues in five test sites. *Computers in Nursing, 15*(1), 23–29.

Gordon, M. (1998). Nursing nomenclature and classification system development. *On-line Journal of Issues in Nursing* [On-line]. Available: www.nursingworld.org/ojin/tpc7/tpc7_1.htm

Grobe, S. J. (1992). Nursing lexicon and taxonomy: Preliminary categorization. In K. C. Lun et al. (Eds.), *Med-Info92: Proceedings of the 7th World Congress on Medical Information.* Amsterdam, Netherlands: Elsevier.

Grulke, C. C. (1995). Seven ways to help a student nurse. *AJN, 96*(60), 24L.

Hayes, B., Norris, J., Martin, K. S., & Androwich, I. (1994). Informatics issues for nursing's future. *Advances in Nursing Science, 16*(4), 71–81.

Iowa Interventions Project. (1993). The NIC taxonomy structure. *Image: Journal of Nursing Scholarship, 25*(3), 187–192.

Johnson, M. (1998). Overview of the Nursing Outcomes Classification (NOC). *On-line Journal of Nursing Informatics, 2*(2) [On-line]. Available: http://cac.psu.edu/~dxm12/OJNI.html

Johnson, M., Bulechek, G., Dochterman, J., Maas, M., & Moorhead, S. (2001). *Nursing diagnoses, outcomes, & interventions, NANDA, NOC, and NIC linkages.* St. Louis, MO: Harcourt Health Sciences.

Johnson, M., & Maas, M. (1998). Implementing the nursing outcomes classification in a practice setting. *Outcomes Management for Nursing Practice, 2*(3), 99–104.

Johnson, M., Maas, M., & Moorhead, S. (Eds.). (2000). *Nursing outcomes classification (NOC)* (2nd ed.). St. Louis, MO: Mosby.

Joint Commission on Accreditation of Healthcare Organizations. (1998). *1998 Hospital accreditation standards.* Oakbrook Terrace, IL: Author.

LaDuke, S. (2000). Spotlight: What you *really* do with this powerful documentation tool. *Nursing2000, 30*(6), 68.

McCloskey, J. C., & Bulechek, G. M. (1994). Standardizing the language for nursing treatments: An overview of the issues. *Nursing Outlook, 42*(2), 56–63.

McCloskey, J. C., & Bulechek, G. M. (1995). Validation and coding of the NIC taxonomy structure. *Image: Journal of Nursing Scholarship, 27*(1), 43–49.

McCloskey, J. C., & Bulechek, G. M. (1998). Nursing interventions classification (NIC): Current status and new directions. *On-line Journal of Nursing Informatics, 2*(2) [On-line]. Available: http://milkman.cac.psu.edu/ndxm12/OJNI.htm

McCloskey, J. C., & Bulechek, G. M. (2000). *Nursing interventions classification (NIC)* (3rd ed.). St. Louis, MO: Mosby.

McCloskey, J. C., & Maas, M. (1998). Interdisciplinary teams: The nursing perspective is essential. *Nursing Outlook, 46*(4), 157–163.

National Committee on Vital and Health Statistics (HCVHS) Hearings on Medical Terminology and Code Development. (1999). *Health care terminology: Nursing outcomes classification, The University of Iowa* [On-line]. Available: http://aspe.os.dhhs.gov/NCVHS/990518t4.htm

National Library of Medicine. (2000). *Fact sheet, UMLS* [On-line]. Available: http://www.nlm.nih.gov/pubs/factsheetsumls.html

North American Nursing Diagnosis Association. (2001). *NANDA Nursing diagnoses: Definitions & classifications 2001–2002.* St. Louis, MO: Author.

Oermann, M. & Huber, D. (1999). Patient outcomes: A measure of nursing's value. *AJN, 99*(9), 40–47.

Ozbolt, J. (1998). *From minimum data to maximum impact: Using clinical data to strengthen patient care* [On-line]. Available: http://cti.itc.virginia.edu/~spt2j/707materials/ozbolt98.htm

Ozbolt, J. G., Fruchtnight, J. N., & Hayden, J. R. (1994). Toward data standards for clinical nursing information. *Journal of the American Medical Informatics Association, 1*(2), 175–185.

Rochman, R. (2000). Are computerized patient records for you? *Nursing2000, 30*(10), 61–62.

The University of Iowa College of Nursing. (2001a). *Strengths of the nursing interventions classification* [On-line]. Available: http://coninfo.nursing.uiowa.edu/nic/strength.htm

The University of Iowa College of Nursing. (2001b). *Nursing outcomes classification overview* [On-line]. Available: http://coninfo.nursing.uiowa.edu/noc/overview.htm

Werley, H. H., & Lang, N. M. (1988). The consensually derived nursing minimum data set: Elements and definitions. In H. H. Werley & N. M. Lang (Eds.), *Identification of the nursing minimum data set* (pp. 402–411). New York: Springer.

White, L. (2001). *Foundations of nursing: Caring for the whole person.* Albany, NY: Delmar.

White, L. (2002). *Basic nursing: Foundations of skills & concepts.* Albany, NY: Delmar.

Wilkinson, J. M. (2000). Nursing diagnosis handbook with NIC interventions and NOC outcomes. Englewood Cliffs, NJ: Prentice Hall.

Resources

American Nursing Informatics Association (ANIA). PMB105, 10808 Foothill Boulevard, Suite 160, Rancho Cucamonga, CA 91730, http://www.ania.org

Center for Nursing Classification, The University of Iowa, College of Nursing, 407 Nursing Building, Iowa City, IA 52242-1121, 319-335-7051, http://www.nursing.uiowa.edu

North American Nursing Diagnosis Association (NANDA). 1211 Locust Street, Philadelphia, PA 19107, 800-647-9002, http://www.nanda.org

CHAPTER 12

REPORTING

LEARNING OBJECTIVES

Upon completion of this chapter, you should be able to:
- *Define key terms.*
- *Compare summary reports, walking rounds, and telephone reports.*
- *Discuss the three types of walking rounds. Describe how to appropriately make a telephone report.*
- *Effectively report to the staff nurse when leaving the unit.*

KEY TERMS

incident report	walking rounds
summary report	

INTRODUCTION

Reporting is the verbal communication of data regarding the client's health status, needs, treatments, outcomes, and responses. A report must summarize the current critical information pertinent to clinical decision making and continuity of care. As with recording, reporting is based on the nursing process, standards of care, and legal and ethical principles. The nursing process provides structure for an organized report, a challenge inherent in verbal communications. In order to verbally communicate an efficient and well-organized report, the nurse must consider the following questions:

- What must be said?
- Why must it be said?
- How must it be said?
- What are the expected outcomes?

Considering these aspects of reporting before communicating the information provides for a concise, organized report.

Another critical element in reporting is listening. Reports require participation from everyone present. When receiving a report, the nurse must focus behaviors to enhance listening skills such as eliminating distractions, putting thoughts and concerns aside, concentrating on those things being said, and not anticipating the presenter's next statements. The reporting process is an integral component of developing effective interpersonal and intrapersonal relationships that promote continuity of client care. Regardless of the type of communication, planned presentation of client data is key to accurate, concise, effective reporting. *Client information reported to other health care providers (e.g. nurse-manager, staff nurses, physician) should also be documented in the client's record.* Summary reports, walking rounds, telephone reports and orders, and incident reports are all types of reporting.

 PROFESSIONAL TIP

Information for Shift Report
1. Client name, room and bed, age, and gender
2. Physician, admission date and diagnosis, and any surgery
3. Diagnostic tests or treatments performed in the past 24 hours; results, if available
4. General status, any significant change in condition
5. New or changed physician's orders
6. Nursing diagnoses and suggested nursing orders
7. Evaluation of nursing interventions
8. Intravenous fluid amounts, last prn medication
9. Concerns about the client

SUMMARY REPORTS

Summary reports outline information pertinent to the client's needs as identified by the nursing process. Summary reports commonly occur either at the change of shift when a new caregiver is involved or when the client is transferred to another area. A summary, or end-of-shift, report should include the following information in the order indicated:

1. Background data obtained from client interactions and assessment of the client's functional health patterns
2. Primary medical and nursing diagnoses and priority problems
3. Identified client risks
4. Recent changes in condition or in treatments (e.g., new medications, elevated temperature)
5. Effective interventions or treatments of priority problems, inclusive of laboratory and diagnostic results (e.g., client's response to pain medication)
6. Progress toward expected outcomes (priority problems, teaching, or discharge planning)
7. Adjustments in the plan of care
8. Client or family complaints

This logical and time-sequenced format follows the nursing process and thus provides structure and organization to the data. In order to provide continuity of care, the new caregiver must receive an accurate, concise report about those things that have happened during the previous shift. Client and family complaints relative to each client should be addressed last, because these situations usually generate questions and discussion.

WALKING ROUNDS

Walking rounds can take the form of nursing rounds, instructor-student rounds, physician–nurse rounds, or multidisciplinary rounds. **Walking rounds** is a reporting method used when the members of the care team walk to each client's room and discuss care and progress with each other and with the client, as shown in Figure 12-1.

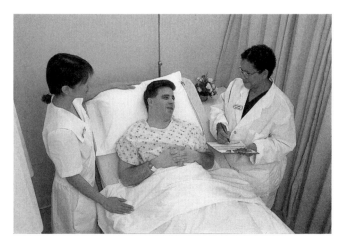

Figure 12-1 Walking Rounds

Nursing rounds are used most frequently by charge nurses as their method of report. During the rounds, the oncoming nurse is introduced to the client and the off-going nurse discusses with the client and the on-coming nurse any changes in the plan of care. Although more time-consuming than a summary end-of-shift report, walking rounds give the nurses and the client the opportunity to evaluate the effectiveness of care together.

Nursing rounds are also used as a teaching method. The instructor introduces the client to the student, and together they discuss the client's care. The instructor can also use this time to appraise the student's observation, communication, and decision-making skills.

Nurse–physician rounds involve the physician and either a staff nurse or the charge nurse. These rounds usually occur daily and provide the nurse, the physician, and the client the opportunity to evaluate the effectiveness of care.

Multidisciplinary rounds, which involve all disciplines, usually occur less frequently than the other types of rounds; primarily because it is difficult to schedule caregivers from all the disciplines for rounds. Multidisciplinary rounds are done most commonly in place of or to supplement case conferences and to discuss discharge planning. Multidisciplinary rounds support the concept of critical pathways and are seen most frequently in facilities that use pathways and/or in large medical teaching institutions.

TELEPHONE REPORTS AND ORDERS

Telephone communications are another way nurses report transfers, communicate referrals, obtain client data, solve problems, and inform a client's family members regarding a change in the client's condition. Nurses are expected to demonstrate telephone courtesy and professionalism when initiating and receiving telephone reports.

When initiating a telephone call, the nurse should organize the information to be reported or received. For example, the nurse should:

- Ensure all lab results are back; if they are not, the nurse should identify in advance those that are missing and should phone the lab or check the computer to ascertain whether other results are available. If phoning the lab, the nurse should spell the client's name and provide the client's medical record number to minimize the chances of receiving results for the wrong client. The nurse should write down those tests that have been performed and the results.
- Review notes and have the client's assessment data readily available, especially any significant data related to abnormal results. If the nurse has not assessed the client, this should be done before telephoning the practitioner; otherwise, the practitioner might ask questions that the nurse is unable to answer.
- Inform the charge nurse or someone else at the nurses' station of plans to place the call, so as to minimize the chances of being interrupted while on the phone.

When placing a call, the nurse should identify herself and state the reason for the call, for example, "this is Ms. White, RN calling Dr. Weng regarding the blood sugar results for Mrs. Koch in room 4203 at Memorial Hospital." The nurse should be brief, listen carefully, and repeat the test results and any orders the physician gives over the phone.

The date and time the phone call was placed, the client data reported by the nurse, the name of the person with whom the nurse spoke, and whether an order was obtained should be recorded accurately in the client's medical record. Rather than charting, "Physician notified, no orders obtained," chart, "Dr. Weng notified by phone, blood sugar 260 mg (drawn by the lab at 1300), orders received and recorded on the physician order sheet." Telephone orders should be charted and the nurses' progress notes updated as soon as possible after the phone call to prevent another caregiver from posting an entry before the telephone orders have been posted.

Figure 12-2 demonstrates the way to write a telephone order on the physician's order sheet: the entry is dated and timed; the order as given by the physician is recorded; and the order is signed beginning with t.o. (telephone order), the physician's name is written, and the nurse's name is signed. If another nurse witnesses the phone order, that nurse's signature should follow the first nurse's signature.

The physician must countersign the order within a time frame specified by the facility's policy. Fax machines have decreased the need for lengthy or complicated telephone orders, both saving time and minimizing errors. The physician should be telephoned to confirm the physician's identity as the initiator of the fax orders. The physician must countersign the fax orders according to agency policy.

INCIDENT REPORTS

Incident reports, or occurrence reports, are used to document any unusual occurrence or accident in the delivery of client care, such as falls or medication errors. Incident reports are not a means of punishing the caregiver; rather, ethical practice requires that the nurse file an incident report to protect the client.

Incident reports are not merely an internal device for the facility; they are required by federal, national, and state accrediting agencies. For legal reasons, nurses are often advised not to document the filing of an incident report in the nurses' notes. As previously discussed, however, a medication error (Grane, 1995) necessitates both an incident report and documentation in the nurses' notes to ensure that the client receives safe care.

PHYSICIAN ORDER SHEET

DATE	HOUR	ORDERS
2/3/02	1420	*Give Demerol 50 mg IM stat.* ————————
		————————*T.O. Dr. Weng/L. White RN*

Figure 12-2 Documenting a Telephone Order

The incident report serves two functions:

- It informs the facility's administration of the incident, thereby allowing risk management personnel to consider changes that might prevent similar occurrences in the future.
- It alerts the facility's insurance company to a potential claim and the need for further investigation.

Each person with firsthand knowledge of the occurrence should fill out and sign a separate report (Figure 12-3). Although the incident report format varies from one facility to another, the following key elements must be addressed when filing a report:

- The date, exact time, and place the nurse discovered the occurrence should be recorded.
- The person(s) involved in the occurrence, including witnesses, should be identified.
- The exact occurrences witnessed by the nurse must be accurately and objectively documented; for example, "Found the client sitting on the floor, client stated that . . . ," rather than "Client fell."
- The exact details of what happened and the consequences for the persons involved must be recorded in time sequence.
- The nurse's actions to provide care and the results of the nurse's assessment for injuries and client complaints should be recorded.
- The supervisor on duty notified and the time and name of the physician notified is recorded. If telephone orders were received from the physician, these should be documented as previously discussed and the orders implemented.
- The nurse should not record personal opinions, judgments, conclusions, or assumptions about what occurred; point blame; or suggest ways to prevent similar occurrences.
- The incident report should be forwarded to the designated person as defined by the facility's policy.

PROFESSIONAL TIP

Documenting an Incident Report

The incident should be factually documented in the nurse's notes, but the notes should not say "incident report filed."

CHRISTUS Health
QUALITY COMMITTEE
VARIANCE REPORT
Medical Record #:
□ Male　□ Female
Name:
Address:
Phone #:

Event Info: *(To Be Completed by Risk Management)*	Event Number _____

FACILITY ID # _____
Persons Involved *(Name, Address, Phone)*

Event Reported By: _____

	Witness	Patient	Employee	Other
	□	□	□	□
	□	□	□	□
	□	□	□	□
	□	□	□	□

1. Event Type:
Variance Occurred to:
□ 01 Patient　□ 03 Student　□ 05 Volunteer
□ 02 Visitor　□ 04 Contract/Registry　□ 06 Physician

Date of Occurrence: _____ / _____ / _____
Time of Occurrence: _____　□ AM/□ PM

2. Body Part *(Check all that apply)*

□ 21 Abdomen	□ 104 Brain	□ 48 Elbow - Left	□ 35 Gastrointestinal	□ 69 Knee - Left	□ 97 Pelvis	□ 06 Teeth - Tooth
□ 71 Ankle - Left	□ 89 Breast - Left	□ 49 Elbow - Right	□ 22 Groin	□ 70 Knee - Right	□ 36 Reproductive Organs	□ 11 Throat
□ 72 Ankle - Right	□ 90 Breast - Right	□ 94 Esophagus	□ 101 Hand - Left	□ 67 Leg - Left	□ 20 Rib	□ 75 Toes
□ 44 Arm - Left	□ 66 Buttock - Left	□ 40 Eye - Left	□ 102 Hand - Right	□ 68 Leg - Right	□ 03 Scalp	□ 34 Urinary Tract
□ 45 Arm - Right	□ 66 Buttock - Right	□ 41 Eye - Right	□ 01 Head	□ 33 Lungs	□ 42 Shoulder - Left	□ 24 Vertebrae
□ 60 Back - Upper (Cervical)	□ 18 Chest	□ 04 Face	□ 32 Heart	□ 05 Mouth	□ 43 Shoulder - Right	□ 46 Wrist - Left
□ 61 Back - Middle (Thoracic)	□ 91 Chin	□ 16 Fingers	□ 63 Hip - Left	□ 10 Neck	□ 02 Skull	□ 47 Wrist - Right
□ 62 Back - Lower (Lumbar)	□ 92 Ear - Left	□ 73 Foot - Left	□ 64 Hip - Right	□ 38 Nervous System	□ 98 Spinal Cord	□ 99 Other
□ 37 Blood Vessels	□ 93 Ear - Right	□ 74 Foot - Right		□ 09 Nose	□ 19 Sternum	□ 39 NA

3. Event Category/Indicator:
(Check one only)

G. Anesthesia
□ 06 Allergic Reaction
□ 10 Arrest
□ 07 Aspiration
□ 02 Dosage
□ 08 Informed Consent
□ 01 Intubation/Extubation
□ 03 Maintaining Airway
□ 05 Medication
□ 09 Monitoring
□ 04 Positioning of Airway
□ 11 Type Unplanned
□ 99 Anesthesia - Other

BE. Behavioral/Conduct
□ 01 AMA or AWOL
□ 04 Assault by Employee
□ 03 Assault by Patient
□ 05 Assault by Third Party
□ 06 Combative
□ 07 Elopement
□ 09 Inappropriate Language
□ 08 Possession Gun/Weapon/
　　 Illegal Substance
□ 10 Self-Inflicted Injuries
□ 11 Self Extubation
□ 02 Suicide Attempt
□ 99 Behavioral/Conduct - Other

W. Blood
□ 01 Adverse Reaction
□ 02 Crossmatch Issue
□ 03 Consent
□ 04 Delay
□ 05 Infiltration
□ 06 Omitted
□ 07 Rate of Flow
□ 08 Site Problem
□ 09 Wrong Patient
□ 10 Wrong Volume
□ 99 Blood - Other

O. Contact With
□ 01 Bodily Fluids
□ 18 Bodily Fluids
□ 12 Chemical
□ 15 Electricity
□ 08 Equipment
□ 16 Fire
□ 21 Flammable Agent
□ 11 Foreign Body
□ 14 Fumes
□ 07 Glass
□ 17 Gloves

□ 104 Hand Tool
□ 20 Latex Product
□ 06 Medical Instruments
□ 02 Needle - Contaminated
□ 03 Needle - Clean
□ 19 Soap
□ 13 Steam/Fluid
□ 22 Sunlight
□ 09 Utensils
□ 99 Contact With - Other

E. Emergency Medicine
□ 02 Admission Issues
□ 13 AMA
□ 10 Death in ER
□ 01 Diagnosis
□ 04 F/U Instructions
□ 06 Inappropriate Treatment
□ 14 Informed Consent
□ 11 Left w/o Treatment
□ 08 Monitoring
□ 12 Return for Same Problem
□ 07 Triage Issues
□ 09 Transfer
□ 99 Emergency - Other

J. Equipment/Supplies/Products
□ 07 Breakage/Damaged
□ 03 Electrical Problem
□ 17 Dietary/Vending
□ 06 Equipment Defect/Malfunction
□ 02 Equipment Failure
□ 20 Implant
□ 18 Pharmaceutical
□ 19 Prosthetic Device
□ 08 Tampered With
□ 04 Unavailable
□ 10 Unsterile
□ 01 Use By Operator
□ 05 Wrong Equipment
□ 99 Equipment/Supplies/Products - Other

If checked, must provide following:
Equipment Disposition _____

Name of Equipment/Product _____
Control # _____
Model # _____
Serial # _____
□ BioMed Notified
□ Device Sequestered

I.　Exposure
□ 08 Chicken Pox
□ 01 Hepatitis
□ 04 Herpes
□ 05 HIV/AIDS
□ 11 Lice
□ 07 Measles
□ 06 Meningitis
□ 09 MRSA
□ 03 Nosocomial
□ 12 Scabies
□ 02 Tuberculosis
□ 10 VRE
□ 99 Exposure - Other

R.　Ingestion
□ 03 Chemical
□ 04 Drug
□ 02 Food Poison
□ 01 Foreign Object in Food
□ 99 Ingestion - Other

C.　Medications & Intravenous
□ 04 Administration Timing
□ 23 Administered to Allergic Patient
□ 08 Adverse Reaction
□ 09 Failure to Order
□ 22 Medication Transcription
□ 10 Narcotic Wastage
□ 06 Omission
□ 01 To Wrong Patient
□ 05 Wrong Medication
□ 03 Dosage
□ 99 Medication - Other

□ 12 IV - Adverse Reaction
□ 07 IV - Infiltration
□ 13 IV - Out of Sequence
□ 14 IV - Rate of Flow
□ 15 IV - Tubing Pulled Out/Broken
□ 16 IV - Wrong/Incomplete Additives
□ 17 IV - Dosage
□ 18 IV - Wrong Patient
□ 19 IV - Wrong Solution
□ 20 IV - Time
□ 21 IV - Other

Type Medication (Check Appropriate
Type(s) Relating to Medication IV Events)
□ 01 Analgesic
□ 02 Antibiotic
□ 03 Anticoagulant
□ 04 Anticonvulsant
□ 05 Antidepressant
□ 06 Antiemetic

□ 07 Antihistamine
□ 08 Antineoplastic
□ 09 Bronchodilator
□ 10 Cardiovascular
□ 11 Contrast Media
□ 12 Diuretic
□ 13 Immunizations
□ 14 Insulin
□ 15 Laxative
□ 16 Narcotics
□ 17 Oxytoxics
□ 18 Radio Nuclides
□ 19 Sedative/Tranq.
□ 20 Vasodilator
□ 21 Vasopressor
□ 99 Other _____

Medication & Dosage Involved:

F.　OB-GYN
□ 06 Apgar <5
□ 07 Contamination
□ 17 C-Section without Consent
□ 03 Timing of Delivery
□ 04 Timing of Performing C-Section
□ 02 Timing of Response
□ 99 Delivery Outside of L&D
□ 05 Fetal Monitor Interpretation
□ 08 Laceration
□ 10 Meconium Aspiration
□ 01 Monitoring
□ 11 Neonatal Injury
□ 12 Precipitous Delivery
□ 13 Return to Delivery Room
□ 14 Unattended Delivery
□ 15 Unusual Condition - Child
□ 16 V-BAC Delivery
□ 99 OB/GYN - Other

Complications:

P.　Security/Crime
□ 01 Arrest Issues
□ 04 Billing Practices
□ 05 Drug Keys
□ 06 Drug Tampering/Narcotic Count
□ 03 Robbery/Assault
□ 99 Security/Crime - Other

COR006 (1/00)　　**Privileged & Confidential**　　**Do Not Copy or Place in Medical File**

(continues)

Figure 12-3 Example of an Incident Report (Courtesy of CHRISTUS Spohn Health System, Corpus Christi, TX)

Iyer and Camp (1999) suggest an additional safeguard for the nurse: writing a brief, accurate description of the incident and keeping it at home. Included in the description should be the details of the incident and the names of the people who were involved, especially if these people can substantiate the nurse's description. Lawsuits may take several years from the time of the incident until the time that the case goes to court; thus, personal notes will help the nurse accurately recall the incident.

A. Slip/Trip/Fall
- ☐ 01 Assisted to Floor
- ☐ 02 Found on Floor
- ☐ 03 On Furniture/Fixed Objects
- ☐ 04 On Liquid/Ice
- ☐ 05 On Stairs/Ramp
- ☐ 06 On Wire or Card

Fall From:
- ☐ A From Bath/Shower
- ☐ B From Bed
- ☐ C From Chair
- ☐ D From Crib/Isolette
- ☐ E From Exam Table
- ☐ F From Toilet
- ☐ G From Wheelchair
- ☐ H From Stretcher/Gurney
- ☐ I From Support Equipment
- ☐ J On Walkway/Parking Lot/Delivery
- ☐ K Slip/Trip w/out Fall
- ☐ L While Ambulating
- ☐ M While Engaged in Recreational Activity
- ☐ N Slip/Trip/Fall - Other

Condition Prior to Fall:
- ☐ 01 Agitated
- ☐ 02 Angry
- ☐ 03 Confused
- ☐ 04 Depressed
- ☐ 05 Oriented/Alert
- ☐ 06 Sedated/Medicated
- ☐ 07 Senile
- ☐ 08 Unconscious
- ☐ 09 Unknown

- ☐ 09 Not Applicable
- ☐ 99 Other _____

Restraints: (In Place Prior to Event)
- ☐ 01 Bed Check
- ☐ 02 Not applicable
- ☐ 021 Unknown
- ☐ 03 Vest
- ☐ 04 Waist
- ☐ 05 Wrist
- ☐ 99 Other _____

Bed Position:
- ☐ 01 Low   ☐ 03 Not Applicable
- ☐ 02 High   ☐ 04 Unknown

Number of Side Rails On Bed:
- ☐ 2   ☐ 4

Side Rails:
- ☐ 01 None   ☐ 04 3 up
- ☐ 02 1 up   ☐ 05 4 up
- ☐ 03 2 up   ☐ 06 Not Applicable
- ☐ 07 Unknown

Call Light In Reach:
- ☐ 01 Yes
- ☐ 02 No

Call Light On:
- ☐ Yes   ☐ No

K. Standard Of Care
- ☐ 06 Documentation/Charting
- ☐ 08 Failure to Notify of Change - Condition

- ☐ 05 Failure to Follow Procedures
- ☐ 09 Monitoring
- ☐ 04 Orientation/Education
- ☐ 07 Physician Response Time
- ☐ 11 Pressure Ulcer
- ☐ 02 Screening/Licensing/Credentialing
- ☐ 03 Staffing
- ☐ 01 Supervision
- ☐ 10 Unauthorized Practice
- ☐ 99 Standard of Care - Other

Q. Struck/Injured By
- ☐ 05 Between Objects
- ☐ 04 By Employee
- ☐ 03 By Patient
- ☐ 06 By Visitor
- ☐ 06 Door
- ☐ 09 During Recreational Activity
- ☐ 07 Elevator
- ☐ 02 Falling/Flying Object
- ☐ 01 Moving Object
- ☐ 99 Struck/Injured By - Other

D. Surgical
- ☐ 18 Canceled Surgery
- ☐ 06 Contamination/Sterile Field
- ☐ 07 Delay in Scheduling/Performing
- ☐ 08 Delay in Closing
- ☐ 05 Informed Consent
- ☐ 13 Injury to Another Organ
- ☐ 04 Instrument/Foreign Body Left in Site
- ☐ 15 Lack of Proper Technique
- ☐ 09 Monitoring
- ☐ 17 Positioning of Patient

- ☐ 12 Postoperative Infection/Complication
- ☐ 10 Prep
- ☐ 03 Sponge/Instrument/Needle Count
- ☐ 16 Unplanned Return to Surgery
- ☐ 11 Unplanned Procedures
- ☐ 01 Wrong Procedure
- ☐ 02 Wrong Patient
- ☐ 99 Surgical - Other

V. Treatment & Procedure
- ☐ 01 Adverse Reaction
- ☐ 02 Application/Removal of Cast/Splint
- ☐ 03 Canceled Procedure
- ☐ 05 Delay
- ☐ 22 Discharged w/heparin/saline lock
- ☐ 04 Informed Consent
- ☐ 06 Invasive Procedure/Placement
- ☐ 07 Missing Specimen
- ☐ 08 Monitoring
- ☐ 09 Omitted
- ☐ 10 Patient Missed Appointment
- ☐ 11 Patient Refusal
- ☐ 12 Positioning
- ☐ 13 Prep Problem
- ☐ 21 Radiation Exposure
- ☐ 14 Repeat Procedure
- ☐ 15 Reporting of Test Results
- ☐ 16 Patient Transfer/Move
- ☐ 17 Wrong Patient
- ☐ 18 Wrong Site
- ☐ 19 Wrong Time
- ☐ 20 Wrong Treatment/Procedure
- ☐ 99 Treatment & Procedures - Other

4. Nature of Injury:
(Check all that apply)
- ☐ 01 Abrasion
- ☐ 04 Abscess
- ☐ 47 AIDS/HIV
- ☐ 06 Amputation
- ☐ 44 Anoxia
- ☐ 28 Avulsion
- ☐ 33 Bite
- ☐ 16 Broken Teeth
- ☐ 08 Burn
- ☐ 30 Bursitis

- ☐ 11 Circulatory Impairment
- ☐ 07 Concussion
- ☐ 17 Contracture
- ☐ 02 Contusion
- ☐ 54 Crushing Injury
- ☐ 29 Dermatitis/Skin Disorder
- ☐ 14 Deterioration on Condition
- ☐ 36 Drowning
- ☐ 55 Enucleation
- ☐ 13 Excessive Blood Loss
- ☐ 56 Exposure
- ☐ 24 Fever
- ☐ 12 Fracture/Dislocation

- ☐ 57 Gun Shot Wound
- ☐ 52 Headache
- ☐ 39 Hearing Impairment
- ☐ 41 Heart Attack
- ☐ 35 Heat Exhaustion/Cramps/Stroke
- ☐ 51 Hematoma
- ☐ 25 Hernia
- ☐ 18 Hypo/Hyper Thermia
- ☐ 58 Ingestion
- ☐ 31 Infection
- ☐ 27 Inflammation
- ☐ 46 Internal Injuries
- ☐ 03 Laceration

- ☐ 49 Multiple Injuries/Whole Body
- ☐ 42 Nervous Disorder
- ☐ 48 No Injury Noted
- ☐ 19 Phlebitis
- ☐ 53 Poison
- ☐ 32 Pressure Ulcer
- ☐ 05 Puncture
- ☐ 20 Reddened Area
- ☐ 43 Respiratory Disorder/Asphyxia/Choking
- ☐ 21 Retained Foreign Object
- ☐ 59 Rupture
- ☐ 22 Seizure
- ☐ 37 Shock (Non-Electrical)

- ☐ 38 Shock (Electrical)
- ☐ 09 Sprain
- ☐ 23 Stillborn
- ☐ 34 Sting
- ☐ 10 Strain
- ☐ 45 Stroke
- ☐ 00 Unknown
- ☐ 40 Visual Impairment
- ☐ 26 Wound Disruption/Drainage
- ☐ 99 Other
- ☐ NA Not Applicable

5. (A) Department (occurrence site) _____ **(B) Department Involved** _____ **(C) Date Reported:** _____ **(D) Time Reported:** _____ AM/PM

6. Primary Location:
- ☐ 01 Crosswalks
- ☐ 12 Bathroom/Patients
- ☐ 14 Bathroom/Public
- ☐ 02 Doorways
- ☐ 03 Driveways
- ☐ 04 Elevator
- ☐ 57 Exam/Treatment Room
- ☐ 05 Foyers/Lobbies
- ☐ 06 Grounds
- ☐ 07 Hallway/Corridor
- ☐ 08 Kitchen
- ☐ 56 Laboratory
- ☐ 52 Nursing Station
- ☐ 09 Offices
- ☐ 51 Parking Garage
- ☐ 11 Parking Lot
- ☐ 10 Pantries/Storeroom
- ☐ 53 Patient Home
- ☐ 13 Patient Room
- ☐ 15 Ramps
- ☐ 55 Receptionist/Clerk Area
- ☐ 17 Snack Bar/Cafeteria
- ☐ 18 Stairs/Stairway
- ☐ 58 Traveling To/From Patient Home
- ☐ 19 Tunnels
- ☐ 20 Waiting Room
- ☐ 16 Walkway/Sidewalk
- ☐ 54 X-Ray Room
- ☐ 21 Other
- ☐ 00 Unknown Site

7. Actions:
(Check all that apply)
- ☐ 01 Ambulance Called
- ☐ 02 Employee Consulted
- ☐ 03 Equipment Modified
- ☐ 04 Emergency Treatment
- ☐ 05 Fire/Emergency Svc Called
- ☐ 07 No Action Taken
- ☐ 08 Notified Family
- ☐ 09 Notified Physician
- ☐ 10 Notified Supervisor
- ☐ 11 Police Called
- ☐ 12 X-Ray Ordered/Taken

8. Does this injury involve (Check only one)
one of these outcomes...
- ☐ 01 Amputation
- ☐ 02 Birth Injury
- ☐ 03 Brain Damage
- ☐ 04 Burn
- ☐ 05 Cosmetic Injury
- ☐ 06 Events Resulting in Disability
- ☐ 07 Foreign Body Retention
- ☐ 08 Fracture
- ☐ 09 HIV Related Occurrence
- ☐ 10 Internal Injuries
- ☐ 16 Interpretation Error, Pathology
- ☐ 17 Interpretation Error, Radiology
- ☐ 11 Kidney Failure
- ☐ 13 Loss of Hearing
- ☐ 12 Loss of Eyesight
- ☐ 14 Loss of Sensation
- ☐ 15 Paraplegic/Quadriplegic Injury
- ☐ 18 Residual Paralysis
- ☐ 19 Septicemia After Admission
- ☐ 20 Unexpected Death

9. Facility Criteria Code _____

Brief narrative description of occurrence (Facts only)

_____
_____
_____
_____
_____
_____
_____

Individual Preparing Report (Print Name): _____   Department Head: _____

Supervisor: _____

Privileged & Confidential   Do Not Copy or Place in Medical File

Figure 12-3 (continued)

Because they may be read by the plaintiff's attorney, the nurse's notes should reflect the same elements as are included in an incident report.

Special attention should be given to documenting falls, because current research shows that client falls constitute 75% to 80% of all incident reports on clinical units (Springhouse, 1999). Client falls are the main reason nurses are sued (Iyer & Camp, 1999).

SUMMARY

- Reporting is verbal communication of data about the client's health status, needs, treatments, outcomes, and responses.
- Summary reports are usually given at the change of shift, when a new care giver is involved, or when the client is transferred to another area.
- Walking rounds include nurse–nurse, nurse–physician, instructor–student, or multidisciplinary rounds. The client is always the center of the reporting and included in it.
- Telephone courtesy and professionalism are expected when initiating or receiving telephone reports.
- Incident reports document any unusual occurrence or accident in the delivery of client care.

Review Questions

1. Summary reports should outline important information about the client as identified by the:
   a. nurse.
   b. physician.
   c. nursing process.
   d. nursing interventions classification.

2. In walking rounds:
   a. the client is included in the report.
   b. all health care givers go to each client.
   c. each client comes to the nurses station.
   d. clients, who are able, walk to the lounge area.

3. Telephone reports should be:
   a. performed daily.
   b. organized and brief.
   c. everything the client says.
   d. undertaken only during the day.

4. Incident reports are filed:
   a. in the administrator's office.
   b. in the front of the client's medical record.
   c. when a client does not respond as expected to a treatment.
   d. when there is any unusual occurrence or accident in the delivery of client care.

CRITICAL THINKING QUESTIONS

1. What are the advantages of summary reports? Of walking rounds?

2. Why are incident reports to be made? Why are they not a part of the client's medical record?

WEB FLASH!

• Search the web for more information on incident reports.
• What can you find on the Internet about reporting?

References/Suggested Readings

Calloway, S. (2001). Preventing communication breakdowns. *RN, 64*(1), 71–74.

Eggland, E. T., & Heinemann, D. S. (1994). *Nursing documentation: Charting, recording, and reporting*. Philadelphia: Lippincott Williams & Wilkins.

Estes, M. E. Z. (2002). *Health assessment & physical examination* (2nd ed.). Albany, NY: Delmar.

Grane, N. B. (1995). Documenting a "harmless" medication error. *Nursing95, 25*(4), 80.

Iyer, P. W., & Camp, N. H. (1999). *Nursing documentation: A nursing process approach* (3rd ed.). St. Louis, MO: Mosby.

Joint Commission on Accreditation of Healthcare Organizations. (1998). *1998 Hospital accreditation standards*. Oakbrook Terrace, IL: Author.

Springhouse. (1998). *Charting made incredibly easy*. Springhouse, PA: Springhouse.

Springhouse. (1999). *Mastering documentation* (2nd ed.). Springhouse, PA: Author.

Stewart, K. (2001). Charting tips: Documenting adverse incidents. *Nursing2001, 31*(3), 84.

White, L. (2001). *Foundations of nursing: Caring for the whole person*. Albany, NY: Delmar.

White, L. (2002). *Basic nursing: Foundations of skills & concepts*. Albany, NY: Delmar.

Appendix A: NANDA Nursing Diagnoses 2001–2002

Activity Intolerance
Risk for Activity Intolerance
Impaired Adjustment
Ineffective Airway Clearance
Latex Allergy Response
Risk for Latex Allergy Response
Anxiety
Death Anxiety
Risk for Aspiration
Risk for Impaired Parent/Infant/Child Attachment
Autonomic Dysreflexia
Disturbed Body Image
Risk for Imbalanced Body Temperature
Bowel Incontinence
Effective Breastfeeding
Ineffective Breastfeeding
Interrupted Breastfeeding
Ineffective Breathing Pattern
Decreased Cardiac Output
Caregiver Role Strain
Risk for Caregiver Role Strain
Impaired Verbal Communication
Decisional Conflict (Specify)
Parental Role Conflict
Acute Confusion
Chronic Confusion
Constipation
Perceived Constipation
Risk for Constipation
Ineffective Coping
Ineffective Community Coping

Readiness for Enhanced Community Coping
Defensive Coping
Compromised Family Coping
Disabled Family Coping
Readiness for Enhanced Family Coping
Ineffective Denial
Impaired Dentition
Risk for Delayed Development
Diarrhea
Risk for Disuse Syndrome
Deficient Diversional Activities
Disturbed Energy Field
Impaired Environmental Interpretation Syndrome
Adult Failure to Thrive
Risk for Falls
Dysfunctional Family Processes: Alcoholism
Interrupted Family Processes
Fatigue
Fear
Deficient Fluid Volume
Excess Fluid Volume
Risk for Deficient Fluid Volume
Risk for Imbalanced Fluid Volume
Impaired Gas Exchange
Anticipatory Grieving
Dysfunctional Grieving
Delayed Growth and Development
Risk for Disproportionate Growth
Ineffective Health Maintenance
Health-Seeking Behaviors (Specify)
Impaired Home Maintenance
Hopelessness
Hyperthermia
Hypothermia
Disturbed Personal Identity
Functional Urinary Incontinence
Reflex Urinary Incontinence
Stress Urinary Incontinence
Total Urinary Incontinence
Urge Urinary Incontinence
Risk for Urge Urinary Incontinence
Disorganized Infant Behavior
Risk for Disorganized Infant Behavior
Readiness for Enhanced Organized Infant Behavior

Ineffective Infant Feeding Pattern
Risk for Infection
Risk for Injury
Risk for Perioperative-Positioning Injury
Decreased Intracranial Adaptive Capacity
Deficient Knowledge
Risk for Loneliness
Impaired Memory
Impaired Bed Mobility
Impaired Physical Mobility
Impaired Wheelchair Mobility
Nausea
Unilateral Neglect
Noncompliance
Imbalanced Nutrition: Less than Body Requirements
Imbalanced Nutrition: More than Body Requirements
Risk for Imbalanced Nutrition: More than Body Requirements
Impaired Oral Mucous Membrane
Acute Pain
Chronic Pain
Impaired Parenting
Risk for Impaired Parenting
Risk for Peripheral Neurovascular Dysfunction
Risk for Poisoning
Post-Trauma Syndrome
Risk for Post-Trauma Syndrome
Powerlessness
Risk for Powerlessness
Ineffective Protection
Rape-Trauma Syndrome
Rape-Trauma Syndrome: Compound Reaction
Rape-Trauma Syndrome: Silent Reaction
Relocation Stress Syndrome
Risk for Relocation Stress Syndrome
Ineffective Role Performance
Bathing/Hygiene Self-care Deficit
Dressing/Grooming Self-care Deficit
Feeding Self-care Deficit
Toileting Self-care Deficit
Chronic Low Self-esteem
Situational Low Self-esteem
Risk for Situational Low Self-esteem
Self-mutilation
Risk for Self-mutilation

Disturbed **S**ensory Perception (Specify: Visual, Auditory, Kinesthetic, Gustatory, Tactile, Olfactory)
Sexual Dysfunction
Ineffective **S**exuality Patterns
Impaired **S**kin Integrity
Risk for Impaired **S**kin Integrity
Sleep Deprivation
Disturbed **S**leep Pattern
Impaired **S**ocial Interaction
Social Isolation
Chronic **S**orrow
Spiritual Distress
Risk for **S**piritual Distress
Readiness for Enhanced **S**piritual Well-Being
Risk for **S**uffocation
Risk for **S**uicide
Delayed **S**urgical Recovery
Impaired **S**wallowing
Effective **T**herapeutic Regimen Management
Ineffective **T**herapeutic Regimen Management
Ineffective Community **T**herapeutic Regimen Management
Ineffective Family **T**herapeutic Regimen Management
Ineffective **T**hermoregulation
Disturbed **T**hought Processes
Impaired **T**issue Integrity
Ineffective **T**issue Perfusion (Specify Type: Renal, Cerebral, Cardiopulmonary, Gastrointestinal, Peripheral)
Impaired **T**ransfer Ability
Risk for **T**rauma
Impaired **U**rinary Elimination
Urinary Retention
Impaired Spontaneous **V**entilation
Dysfunctional **V**entilatory Weaning Response
Risk for Other-Directed **V**iolence
Risk for Self-Directed **V**iolence
Impaired **W**alking
Wandering

Appendix B: Abbreviations, Acronyms, and Symbols

a̅	before
a.c.	before meals
ad lib	freely, as desired
AEB	as evidenced by
AJN	*American Journal of Nursing*
ANA	American Nurses Association
bid	twice a day
BP	blood pressure
c	cup
c̅	with
C	Celsius
C & S	culture and sensitivity
cap	capsule
CBE	charting by exception
cc	cubic centimeter
cm	centimeter
COBRA	Comprehensive Omnibus Budget Reconciliation Act
CPR	computerized patient record
dc	discontinue
dL	deciliter
dr	dram
DRG	diagnosis-related group
elix	elixir
F	fahrenheit
g	gram
g/dL	grams per deciliter
gr	grain
gtt	drop
gtt/min	drops per minute
h	hour(s)

Hct	hematocrit
Hgb	hemoglobin
HIS	hospital information system
HR	heart rate
h.s.	hour of sleep
I&O	intake and output
IM	intramuscular
IV	intravenous
JCAHO	Joint Commission on Accreditation of Healthcare Organizations
kg	kilogram
KVO	keep vein open
L	liter
lb	pound
L/min	liters per minute
LOC	level of consciousness
LP/VN	licensed practical/vocational nurse
LPN	licensed practical nurse
LVN	licensed vocational nurse
MAR	medication administration record
mcg (or μg)	microgram
mEq	milliequivalent
mEq/L	milliequivalents per liter
mg	milligram
mL	milliliter
NA	not applicable
NANDA	North American Nursing Diagnosis Association
NCLEX-PN®	National Council Licensure Examination—Practical Nurse
NCLEX-RN®	National Council Licensure Examination—Registered Nurse
NFLPN	National Federation of Licensed Practical Nurses, Inc.
NG	nasogastric
NIC	Nursing Interventions Classification
NIS	nursing information system
NMDS	nursing minimum data set
NOC	Nursing Outcomes Classification
NPO	nil per os, Latin for "nothing by mouth"
NS	normal saline
O_2	oxygen
oz	ounce
$\overline{p}$	after
P	pulse

p.c.	after meals
PCA	patient-controlled analgesia
PIE	problem, implementation, evaluation
po	per os, Latin for "by mouth"
POMR	problem-oriented medical record
POR	problem-oriented record
PPS	prospective payment system
PRO	peer review organization
q	quaque, Latin for "every"
qd	every day
qh	every hour
qid	four times a day
qod	every other day
qs	quantity sufficient
q2h	every 2 hours
R (Resp)	respiration
RBC	red blood count
RN	registered nurse
ROM	range of motion
R/T	related to
RT	rectal temperature
s̄	without
SOAP	subjective data, objective data, assessment, plan
SOAPIE	subjective data, objective data, assessment, plan, implementation, evaluation
SOAPIER	subjective data, objective data, assessment, plan, implementation, evaluation, revision
s̄s̄	one half
T	temperature
tab	tablet
Tbsp	tablespoon
t.i.d.	three times a day
t.o.	telephone order
TPR	temperature, pulse, respirations
tsp	teaspoon
U	unit
UA	routine urinalysis
U/L	unit per liter
UMLS	Universal Medical Language System
VS	vital signs
WNL	within normal limits
wt	weight

Appendix C: Answers to Review Questions

Chapter 1

1. **b.** It is a circular, dynamic process.
2. **b.** implementation.
3. **c.** National Federation of Licensed Practical Nurse's *Standards of Care.*

Chapter 2

1. **d.** temperature 102°F.
2. **a.** nausea.
3. **b.** focused.
4. **c.** Maslow's hierarchy of needs.

Chapter 3

1. **c.** about a client's responses to health problems.
2. **c.** diagnostic label.
3. **a.** etiology.
4. **d.** desires to attain a higher level of wellness.

Chapter 4

1. **c.** client's nursing diagnoses, goals, expected outcomes, and the nursing interventions.
2. **b.** client needs regarding referral agencies
3. **d.** client behavior, measurement criteria, conditions under which the behavior occurs, and target date.
4. **a.** may be handwritten or computer generated.

Chapter 5

1. **b.** delegating some interventions.
2. **a.** cognitive skills.
3. **c.** constitutes a legal record of care to the client.

Chapter 6

1. **c.** during each aspect of the nursing process.
2. **b.** evaluates the quality of client care.

Chapter 7

1. **d.** presents in a logical fashion the care provided by nurses.
2. **c.** accountability and responsibility.
3. **b.** legible, neat writing.
4. **a.** physician.
5. **a.** nurse.

Chapter 8

1. **c.** reflect the nursing process.
2. **d.** medication administration record.
3. **c.** have one line drawn through it.
4. **b.** approved by the facility may be used.

Chapter 9

1. **b.** is the most flexible of all methods.
2. **c.** the plan of care and interventions are recorded together.
3. **b.** problem.
4. **a.** data, action, response.
5. **d.** follows the components of the nursing process.

Chapter 10

1. **a.** a reference.
2. **d.** make it easy to track changes in a client's condition.
3. **a.** personal care flow sheet, MAR, and I&O form.
4. **b.** itemizes client instructions.

Chapter 11

1. **b.** computerized charting.
2. **c.** label, definition, and activities.
3. **d.** evaluate the effects of nursing interventions.

Chapter 12

1. **c.** nursing process.
2. **a.** the client is included in the report.
3. **b.** organized and brief.
4. **d.** when there is any unusual occurrence or accident in the delivery of client care.

Glossary

Actual Nursing Diagnosis Indicates that a problem exists; it is composed of the diagnostic label, related factors, and signs and symptoms.

Advance Directive Written instructions about an individual's health care preferences regarding life-sustaining measures that guide family members and health care professionals as to those treatment options that should or should not be considered in the event that the individual is unable to decide.

Analysis Breaking down the whole into parts that can be examined.

Assessment The first step in the nursing process that includes the systematic collection, verification, organization, interpretation, and documentation of client data.

Assessment Model A framework that provides a systematic method for organizing data.

Assign Give a specific nursing task to assistive (unlicensed) personnel capable of competently performing the task.

Assumptions Those beliefs or attitudes that one takes for granted in a situation that requires action or resolution; they are the things that one accepts as "given."

Bias A personal judgment or inclination.

Charting by Exception Only deviations from pre-established norms are documented.

Collaborative Problem Certain physiologic complications that nurses monitor to detect onset or changes in status. Nurses manage collaborative problems using physician-prescribed and nursing-prescribed interventions to minimize the complications of the events (Carpenito, 2000).

Comprehensive Assessment Gathers client information through a complete health history, physical examination, a review of psychosocial aspects of the client's health, client's perception of health, presence of health risk factors, and the client's coping pattern; a baseline against which changes in the client's health status can be measured.

Critical Pathway A comprehensive, preprinted interdisciplinary standard plan of care reflecting the ideal course of treatment for the average client with a given diagnosis or procedure, especially those with relatively predictable outcomes.

Database Information about the client prior to entering the health care system; the information foundation against which changes in the client's health status is measured.

Data Clustering Process of putting data together in order to identify areas of the client's problems and strengths.

Defining Characteristics Collected data, also known as signs and symptoms, subjective and objective data, or clinical manifestations.

Delegation Process of transferring a select nursing task to another licensed individual who is competent to perform that specific task.

Dependent Nursing Intervention Those actions that require an order from a physician or another health care professional.

Discharge Planning Preparing for the client's needs after discharge.

Documentation Written evidence of interactions between and among health professionals, clients, their families, and health care organizations; administration of tests, procedures, treatments, and client education; and results of or client's response to, diagnostic tests and interventions (Eggland & Heinemann, 1994).

Etiology The related cause or contributor to the problem; identified in the complete NANDA diagnosis description.

Evaluation The fifth step in the nursing process involves determining whether the client goals have been met, partially met, or not met.

Expected Outcome A detailed, specific statement that describes the methods through which the goal will be achieved, including aspects such as direct nursing care, client teaching, and continuity of care.

Focus Charting Documentation method that uses a column format to chart data, actions, and response (DAR).

Focused Assessment An assessment that is limited in scope in order to concentrate on a particular need or health care concern or on potential health care risks.

Goal An aim, intent, or end; broad statements that describe the intended or desired change in the client's condition or behavior.

Health History A review of the client's functional health patterns prior to the current contact with the health care system.

Implementation Execution of the nursing care plan derived during the planning phase.

Independent Nursing Intervention Nursing actions initiated by the nurse that do not require direction or an order from another health care professional.

Incident Report Used to document any unusual occurrence or accident in the delivery of client care, such as falls or medication errors.

Informed Consent A competent client's ability to make health care decisions based on full disclosure of the benefits, risks, and potential consequences of a recommended treatment plan and of alternative treatments including no treatment, and the client's agreement to the treatment as indicated by the client's signing a consent form.

Initial Planning Development of a preliminary plan of care by the nurse who performs the admission assessment.

Interdependent Nursing Intervention Those nursing actions that are implemented in a collaborative manner by the nurse in conjunction with other health care professionals.

Kardex A summary worksheet reference of basic client care information, traditionally not part of the medical record.

Long-term Goal An objective statement outlining the desired resolution of the nursing diagnosis over a longer period of time (weeks or months); focus on problem or nursing diagnosis.

Medical Diagnosis Clinical judgment by the physician that identifies or determines a specific disease, condition, or pathologic state.

Narrative Charting The traditional method of nursing documentation is a chronologic account written in paragraphs describing the client's status, interventions and treatments, and the client's response to them.

Nursing Audit A method of evaluating the care provided to clients by reviewing client records after discharge.

Nursing Care Plan A written guide that organizes data about a client's care into a formal statement of the strategies that will be implemented to help the client achieve optimal health.

Nursing Diagnosis A clinical judgment about individual, family, or community responses to actual or potential health problems/life processes. A nursing diagnosis provides the basis for selection of nursing interventions to achieve outcomes for which the nurse is accountable (NANDA, 2001).

Nursing Intervention An action performed by the nurse that helps the client achieve results specified by the goals and expected outcomes.

Nursing Interventions Classification (NIC) A comprehensive standardized language for nursing interventions organized in a three-level taxonomy.

Nursing Minimum Data Set Elements that should be contained in clinical records and abstracted for studies on the effectiveness and costs of nursing care.

Nursing Outcomes Classification (NOC) A taxonomy of client outcomes for nursing care using comprehensive standardized language.

Nursing Process A systematic method of planning and providing care to clients.

Objective Data (signs) Observable and measurable information that is obtained through both standard assessment techniques and the results of laboratory and diagnostic testing.

Ongoing Assessment An assessment that includes systematic monitoring and observation related to a specific problem.

Ongoing Planning Continuous updating of the client's plan of care as new information is gathered and evaluated.

PIE Charting Streamlined documentation that evolved using only Problem, Intervention, and Evaluation.

Planning The third step of the nursing process; includes both the formulation of guidelines that establish the proposed course of nursing action in the resolution of nursing diagnoses and the development of the client's plan of care.

Point-of-Care Charting A computerized documentation system that allows health care providers to have immediate access to client information.

Potential Complication The first two words of a collaborative problem statement.

Primary Source The major provider of information about a client, generally the client.

Problem-oriented Medical Record Focuses on the client's problems and employs a structured, logical format called SOAP charting.

Process A series of steps or acts that lead to accomplishment of some goal or purpose.

Protocol A series of standing orders or procedures that should be followed under certain specific conditions.

Risk Nursing Diagnosis (potential problem) Indicates that a problem does not yet exist, but that special risk factors are present.

Secondary Sources Data other than that given by the client including family members, laboratory and diagnostic tests, other health care providers, and medical records.

Short-term Goal An objective statement outlining the desired resolution of the nursing diagnosis over a short period of time, usually a few hours or days (less than a week); focus on etiology of nursing diagnosis.

Source-oriented Charting A narrative recording, on separate sheets, by each member (source) of the health care team.

Specific Order An order written in a client's medical record or nursing care plan by a physician or nurse especially for that individual client; it is not used for any other client.

Standing Order A standardized intervention written, approved, and signed by a physician that is kept on file within health care agencies to be used in predictable situations or in circumstances requiring immediate attention.

Subjective Data (symptoms) Information from the client's (sometimes family's) point of view that includes feelings, perceptions, and concerns.

Summary Report Information pertinent to the client's needs as identified by the nursing process shared verbally.

Synthesis Putting data together in a new way.

Variance Goals not met or interventions not performed according to the established time frame.

Walking Rounds A reporting method used when the members of the care team walk to each client's room and discuss care and progress with each other and the client.

Wellness Nursing Diagnosis Indicates the client's expression of a desire to attain a higher level of wellness in some area of function.

Index

Note: Page numbers in **bold type** reference non-text material.